Love, Laughter, & a High Disregard for Statistics

Sue Buchanan

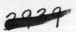

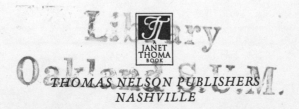

A JANET THOMA BOOK

THOMAS NELSON PUBLISHERS
NASHVILLE

Unless otherwise noted, all Scripture quotations are from THE NEW KING JAMES VERSION of the Bible. Copyright © 1979, 1980, 1982, Thomas Nelson, Inc., Publishers. `

Scripture quotations taken from the HOLY BIBLE: NEW INTERNATIONAL VERSION (R) are marked (NIV) in the text. Copyright © 1973, 1978, 1984 by International Bible Society. Used by permission of Zondervan Publishing House. All rights reserved.

Published in Nashville, Tennessee, by Janet Thoma Books, a division of Thomas Nelson, Inc., Publishers, and distributed in Canada by Word Communications, Ltd., Richmond, British Columbia, and in the United Kingdom by Word (UK), Ltd., Milton Keynes, England.

Published in association with the Literary Agency of Alive Communications, P.O. Box 49068, Colorado Springs, CO 80949.

Library of Congress 93-86889   ISBN 0-8407-4423-4

Printed in the United States of America

2 3 4 5 6 — 98 97 96 95 94

Contents

To Wayne, of course.

Acknowledgments

Thank you!

My family! Wayne, the good guy in the book, who thinks I can accomplish anything and is my greatest support. Dana who encouraged me each step of the way and was always available to talk things over. Melinda (who has legally changed her name to Mary Jane in honor of my mother), for going beyond the call of duty in straightening the house, loading the dishwasher, and doing laundry while I was busy on the computer.

Author Jerry Jenkins, who said, "You do have a book in you!" then cheered me each step of the way. And he put me in touch with his literary agent, Rick Christian.

Rickly Christian of Alive Communications not only helped me learn to write (Hey, Sue, have you ever thought about using conversation in your writing?), but he also helped me find the best publisher for my book.

Joy MacKenzie and Peggy Benson! Joy and Peggy's job was to keep me from embarrassing myself with my publisher. In fact, Joy saved them hours of work by going through each of my chapters and offering suggestions. She even taught me there was a method to punctuation. Joy also came up with the title.

Rose Ann Miller, director of the Institute at Baptist Hospital, who was my "authority" on most medical issues, including cancer hotline numbers and plastic surgery issues. One weekend she let me use her summer home in the woods where I did some of my most intense writing (and fishing).

Larry Stone and Murray and Donna Fisher and Gloria Gaither who never stopped encouraging me and helped me through the problems that come from being a first-time author.

Jon Davis, my brother who helped me with the computer. Although he hasn't always been kind, I'm still thanking him. He said the length of my fingernails rendered me useless to society, much less a keyboard. He asked if I had software and I said it's none of your business what I buy at Victoria's Secret. And he never lets me forget about the night I called to tell him my computer had stopped and no matter what I tried nothing worked. After fifteen minutes of ineffective instructions by phone, he drove to my house. He turned the little knob with the picture of the sun over it (the brightness control) and voila! it worked.

To my family: Becky Davis, Joe Davis, Carolyn Davis, and Sarah Dunn.

My Sunday night group, who loves me, prays for me, laughs with me, and encourages me: Paul Keckley, Rhonda Keckley, Jimmy Hodges, Lynn Hodges, Joy MacKenzie, Bob MacKenzie, Marsha Blackburn, Chuck Blackburn, Evelyn Allen, John Yarborough, Betsy Yarborough, Tommy Thompson, Phyllis Thompson.

Gloria Gaither

Laura Emery, Joy Williams, Bonnie Shafer, The Hipple Cancer Institute, Dr. Martin J. Murphy, Jr., Dr. Ralph Parchment, Dr. Connie Erickson-Miller, Vanderbilt University Breast Center, Dr. Alan Winfield, Dr. Marvin Burnett and staff at HOA, Kate Rupert. And finally, my cats—Jazz and Dizz.

Chapter 1

Red
and Pink
and Purple

My husband climbed into my hospital bed with me. His arm went around my shoulder as his free hand stroked my face and neck. He caressed my arm and traced the veins in my wrist and then each finger. As his dear, familiar hands roamed my body he carefully avoided the place he usually touched first. My breasts. Breasts big enough to evoke teasing from my close friends.

Years earlier, my friend Peggy's four-year-old son Patrick, who was the same age as my Mindy, had climbed on my lap, looked me over, and said, "You sure do have bosoms!" A few days later my husband, Wayne, and I joined Peggy and her husband, Bob, for dinner. As we got out of our respective cars in the parking lot of Jimmy Kelly's restaurant, the two of them shouted in unison, "You sure do have bosoms!" I cringed and glanced around, hoping no one heard. My family had never joked about such things. In fact as I was growing up, my father referred to my bra as "that undergarment you wear." Wayne and I had recently moved to Nashville from a rather stuffy community in the north where breasts or bosoms, for that matter, weren't discussed in public. At least not in our circle of friends.

Everybody in the parking lot of Kelly's heard, including the doorman, the valet, and an elderly couple getting out of a cab, and everyone was laughing. I felt awkward, but managed a tenuous smile, hoping to show what a good sport I was. The next thing I knew, I had wholeheartedly joined them *and* my husband, in their belly laughs. For the first time in my life, I was laughing at my top-heavy figure. We all laughed just as hard on another night, in another restaurant, when Bob looked in the direction of my chest and said, "You seem tired; sit down and get a load off your feet!"

Not only could we tease about my breasts, but as our friendship developed, so did our ability to find more opportunities to joke about each other's flaws. "Distinguishing characteristics," we called them. When we went swimming, we laughed about Bob's puny body and the "one, lonesome hair" on his chest. There was always a good-natured dig at my husband's weight problem: "Pull up a couple of chairs and sit down!" In the same manner, we joked about Peggy's "Bugs Bunny" teeth. The fact that her teeth protruded was one of the reasons she was so cute, in my opinion. They were, and are, such a vital part of her. So very *Peggy*. Likewise, even though I was embarrassed by the size of them, I realized my breasts were an essential element of my *Sue*-ness. They were the essence of my equilibrium and balance and of my lovemaking. One caress made my heart pound and my body tingle.

That was before the operation. Now there was nothing to touch but a bandage six inches thick, which encased my upper torso like a mummy. It was so thick, I had nothing to wear over it, only the ugly hospital gown designed to fit any physique, male or female, fat or thin, tall or short—or someone with only one breast.

Looking down at the faded unibody rag, my mind ached as I thought of never again being able to wear the silky, low-cut gowns I loved so much. I was pained to think how this would affect my husband who, in our first year of marriage, jokingly threatened to throw me on the floor if I ever came to bed in "one of those" flannel nightgowns. Even though he was joking, I remembered how distastefully he spat out the words, much the way he would describe "*one of those* wretched sopranos" or "*one of those* dreadful little barking dogs." Lying there in the hospital, I was sure I'd never again enjoy doing what felt so very good: crawling between the sheets and feeling the pleasurable closeness of skin against skin.

That's exactly what I was thinking. Not about cancer or what I might face as a result of this awful disease: months of sickening chemotherapy; burns from radiation; the loss of hair or maybe even my eyebrows and fingernails; or the possibility of dying at the hands of this cruel killer. I now was only dealing with the unsightly loss of my breast, a part of my body that had been important to me since I was thirteen.

Maybe it was because I grew up during the Marilyn Monroe era. Whatever the reason, breasts were on everyone's mind at Charleston, West Virginia's Woodrow Wilson Junior High School in 1948. Boys whispered about them and girls wanted them. Even then we sensed they were symbols of our femininity. Our primary concerns were, "When will I have them?" "How big will they be?" and "Will it happen overnight?"

The questions were answered one morning when I woke up, turned over on my stomach in bed, and had the strangest feeling I'd rolled on top of the cat. Since I didn't hear the prerequisite "Mrr-ye-ow!" I reached down to feel what other obtrusion might be present and was profoundly surprised to discover it was me—two mounds of me that weren't there before. One day I was flat as a pancake; the next, my mother hustled me off to Stone and Thomas Department Store where I was fitted (in those days it was almost like being fitted for shoes) in a bra, size 32B. Some kids skipped the second or third grade; I skipped an A cup.

The day we purchased bras, my mother bought me a hunter green sweater and color-coordinated plaid skirt. Giggling as I stood sideways in front of the mirror, we decided I looked pretty good and pretty grown up. The next day, in my new outfit, I gave a campaign speech to my seventh grade class, stating my promises if elected class president. Afterward, as I made my way to the back of the auditorium, I saw Darryl Riley take a quick glance around to see if anyone was watching. Then he stepped toward my brand new anatomy with both hands open and a wicked look in his seventh grader eyes, and proceeded to give me the quickest "squeeze" in history. From that moment on, I had mixed feelings about breasts.

In junior high school, most girls—if they had breasts at all—had compact, pert little breasts. I soon graduated from a B to a C cup, which was not at all becoming on my otherwise undeveloped, straight-as-a-stick figure. No one had breasts the size of mine, not even the teachers. My endowment was sheer torture on my young, peer-pressured psyche, and I would have swapped for a set of compact little breasts in an instant.

In gym class I thought of myself as a freak in the institutional, one-piece, blue cotton uniform we had to wear. The outfit was baggy over my shapeless hips and the elastic kept losing its grip on what was supposed to be the wide part of my toothpick legs. The biggest problem was the top. It stretched tightly over my chest and gaped wide between snaps. My breasts bounced right along with the basketball and felt sore for hours afterwards.

Nothing was worse, though, than taking a shower at the end of class. It was the rule: Strip naked and be monitored under the full force of the water. The girls who did the monitoring were invariably the teacher's pets, cheerleader-types with tan bodies and—you guessed it—compact, pert little breasts! Overwhelmed with insecurities, I *died* each time I was forced to undress and parade through the shower.

By the time I went to college I was a 32 Double D, once again skipping a cup size, and I'd come to think of my top-heavy figure as acceptable, even pleasing—to me, as well as to others. I remember one spring night, a group of the guys sat at the foot of the stairway in the girls' dorm, and as we came down to dinner, they whispered and laughed and looked us over from head to toe. We, of course, wanted in on their secret, so we questioned, only to discover they were assembling the "perfect woman" from our various body parts. This was before the women's movement, light years before any of us could spell or even define the word *chauvinist*.

We kept prying and then laughed along when we found

out the ideal body consisted of Marge Sweet's angelic face, Marjorie Johnson's thick shining hair, JayCee Matt's cute shapely legs, Janice Woodring's backside, and my front side. Although no one said the word "breasts" aloud in those days, they beat around the bush with enough "Sue's—*you know!*" that any fool could figure out what part of *me* completed their jigsaw puzzle of perfection.

Now one of those "perfect" breasts was gone forever. On the sixth floor of Baptist Hospital in Nashville, Tennessee, my husband and I were alone. Visitors had been coming and going all day, but it was quiet for the moment. Wayne hadn't left my side: fluffing my pillows, holding the straw while I sipped water, stewing about too many visitors, and making jokes when the conversation became overly serious.

As we lay there, our bodies pressed together, Wayne reminded me that he'd taken care of me for almost twenty-five years and assured me that he would continue to do that, no matter what. However, as I watched him watching me, I wondered if those were just empty words to make me feel better. He said he'd love me, this man who had so wholeheartedly enjoyed my breasts, but how could I be so sure he'd love just half of me?

Wayne and I have always loved each other, but there were times we didn't much *like* each other, and a couple of times we thought we couldn't go on. During the downs, I often quoted my father: "Okay, now, let's just snap out of it!" or "We've mulligrubbed long enough now!" or "It's time to bounce back!"

Years before in a dark, despairing moment, I had stood on the balcony of a hotel, high above Philadelphia, and fought a compelling urge to jump, to end my feeling of utter desolation. I knew I was high enough to ensure a fatal fall, but fortunately I reasoned that my two daughters couldn't make it without a mother or survive the stigma of such an act. Eventually, my husband loved me back from the edge.

Many years after that, not so very long ago, in fact, Wayne wrote me a letter during a bad time, saying why we *should not* divorce. He listed such things as forsaken dreams and memories, the hurt it would bring our daughters, the regrets we'd harbor, and then he reassured me of his love despite our conflicts. "Love is strong enough to get us through," he wrote.

Could he offer the same reassurance now that my body was repulsive? Could he once again love me back from the edge of despair? Perhaps equally important, would I give him the chance?

Silently we lay—side by side in each other's arms, engulfed in our own private thoughts. Above our heads hung twelve helium-filled balloons in various shades of red and pink and purple. Trailing from them, just low enough to touch, were the ribbons, the kind that crinkle and curl when scraped with scissors, the kind my mother-in-law, Mom Buchanan, used to tie up her packages. As Wayne and I finally began to talk about the events that brought us to this moment, we fingered the ribbons, pulling a balloon toward us and letting go, pulling and letting go. We watched it bounce against the ceiling, just as our emotions, and even our prayers, seemed to be doing. One thing was obvious; the balloons had far more resiliency than we did at that moment, maybe more than we could ever hope for again.

2

Tomorrow Is Just a Day Away

I don't remember when I found the lump. In fact, there never really was a lump, just a thickening in the lower left quadrant of my left breast. When I was in the tub and my fingers were soapy, I felt it. Then later, feeling nothing, I could talk myself out of the possibility.

Long before I was even able to feel the thickening, I had begun to have a hurting. Actually, it was more like a heaviness, an uneasiness, in my breast. I tried to put it out of my mind, but the feeling nagged me, like the memory of a nightmare. Neither could I ignore magazine articles that told me my chances of having breast cancer were considerably higher than normal because the disease ran in my family. The odds were against me: Mother had recently had a mastectomy.

Terrified by the grim statistics, I finally called my gynecologist's office. The receptionist sensed the urgency in my voice as I described my problem and scheduled an appointment that very afternoon. Within hours, I was in the examination room, slipping into a white, sterile-smelling cotton gown.

"Put the opening toward the front, just opposite what you would think," the tall, grayhaired nurse instructed. As I climbed onto the examining table, I glanced at the stirrups and took comfort in knowing that today at least, I'd be spared that particular contortion. I fanned through an outdated, dog-eared magazine I'd picked up in the waiting room, the only kind doctors ever stock. I couldn't concentrate.

My stomach felt queasy. I glanced at my watch. Then my eyes followed the straight line of pictures around the perimeter of the room. Ducks, perfect ducks, all headed in the same direction, all nearly identical, all framed alike in narrow black frames with gray linen mats. "Quack doctor's office," I muttered to myself, unable to fathom why anyone would want so many ducks that looked so alike. I could only hope the doctor would consider me as a unique individual, different from the long line of patients who had preceded and would follow me, each with distinct needs and concerns.

If I had to wait much longer, I'd amuse myself by removing the pictures and hanging them upside down. My children and I had done that very thing, years ago, while waiting for our pediatrician. (What do you do with two little girls stripped down to their panties, who know the doctor has decided their fate—a needle in the bottom—before he even comes through the door?)

"Help yourself to the coloring book and crayons," the nurse had said and gestured to the bottom shelf of the supply table. We had every intention of coloring. We were poised and ready, but there wasn't an inch of clean space anywhere. The book was scribbled full!

"What *can* we color on?" I had asked. Two little-girl voices shouted the obvious answer: "The walls?" I was tempted! Then I spotted the big jar of tongue depressors, grabbed a handful, and for the next fifteen minutes we drew little people pictures on them and lined them up on every available surface. Still no doctor. I looked at my watch and realized we'd been waiting at least forty-five minutes. I'd like to blame what happened next on the children, but to be honest it was my idea, not to mention the fact that the girls couldn't possibly have *reached* the pictures and diplomas displayed on the walls, much less manipulated them to an upside down position. We never again had to wait for Dr. Harvey!

Suddenly my mind snapped to the present as "Doctor Duck" marched through the door, his nurse right at his heels.

We exchanged brief greetings and he introduced "*Maawgret*" (*Margaret* in any language other than southern aristocratic), whom I'd met on many other occasions. Still her presence always seemed to need explaining.

"*Maawgret* will be assisting me." I glanced her way, wondering if the two of them knew I realized she was his star witness if a patient should decide to bring litigation against him for an impropriety.

"What seems to be the problem?" he asked.

I looked at him for a long moment, trying to summon my best business voice. I swallowed hard, but the words came out in four awkward gulps: "Lump in my breast."

"Let's have a look," he said, gently opening my gown. I pointed to my left breast. For the next few minutes, I stared at his thinning scalp as he examined my breast thoroughly, grinding his fingers, it seemed, into every millimeter of flesh. The nurse, bent slightly at the waist, tilted her head this way and that as she followed the movements of his hands.

"Does this hurt?" he asked as his fingers dug deep into the soft tissue.

"Uncomfortable, yes. Hurt, no," I replied.

"How about this?"

I shook my head.

"And this?"

"No."

Next, he was squeezing my nipple. As he squeezed and released, squeezed and released, he fired rapid questions.

"Any discharge?"

"No."

"Bleeding?"

"No."

"Pain here?"

I shook my head.

"Here?" he asked as his hand moved off target center.

"No."

"Puckering? Change of contour?"

"None of the above."

With each question his nurse watched my eyes carefully.

Almost before I'd formed my answer, her head would bob as if it were on a spring, as though she was trying to beat me to my answer. Maybe every other woman that day had said no to the questions and she expected the same from me. I suddenly felt I was on some sort of conveyor belt—that it didn't matter what I said because my diagnosis would automatically be identical to patients A, B, and C, who preceded me.

I looked at the ducks while the doctor checked my right breast as thoroughly as he had the left. When he finished, he buried his head in my chart and in his doctor-style mumble reviewed my gynecological history without seeming to take a breath: Two children, seven years on the pill; two lumpectomies; IUD lodged in the wall of the uterus and suspected pregnancy; hysterectomy; hormone tablets. He glanced at me as though we shared a secret. "They did the trick, didn't they?" he asked. "The hormone pills."

"No more hot flashes. And my sex life improved . . . considerably!" I answered.

A few more mumbles, then he shut the folder and suggested I dress and join him in the next room. I knew his procedure well; the examining room was for examining, the office next door was for discussing his findings. He always used colorful illustrations with his explanations. I'd seen his pictures of healthy ovaries and diseased ovaries, healthy uteruses and diseased uteruses, likewise fallopian tubes and every other healthy and diseased gynecological probability. The business woman in me liked this *modus operandi*. It seemed much more humane and dignified to have a discussion fully clothed, sitting eye to eye across a desk than as some doctors did it, pontificating while I lay on my back on the examining table.

I stood and reached for my clothes. I pulled my bra out from under my folded blouse, under because that's where my mother had told me to put it. "It's not ladylike for your underwear to be in plain open sight," she had always said. I put on my bra and buttoned my blouse, comforting myself with the fact I'd seen no worry in the doctor's eyes. Neither had I felt any sense of urgency, which surely would have been present were my breast or life in danger.

Minutes later in his cluttered office, he reached for the ever-present medical illustrations. "This is a healthy breast," he said, pointing with his pencil. "And here we have a diseased breast." He carefully shuffled the pictures, allowing me to examine them closely. He then handed me a third illustration. "This shows fibrous cysts or tumors. They aren't malignant, but they certainly are bothersome and can easily be misdiagnosed. Some studies indicate they're *pre*cancerous. That is, they could eventually turn into cancer."

The pictures looked alike to me. All three breasts were mottled, only the shadings seemed different, like the same photograph printed at different exposures. I waited impatiently. I wanted to ask, "Do I or don't I have a problem? Answer yes or no!"

"You just happen to have very lumpy breasts, and we'll have to watch them. But I don't think you have a thing to worry about," he continued with a smile in his voice. "Just to be sure, though, I'll put you in touch with a breast specialist." He jotted a name on a prescription pad and handed it to me as he pushed himself back from the desk.

I thanked him and stood to leave. Then I remembered one more thing. "I know I told you my breast didn't hurt when you examined it. It didn't, not then. However, it does hurt most all the time. I just can't pinpoint *where*."

"Well, that's probably a good sign," he said, ushering me out. "There's rarely, if ever, *any* pain with breast cancer."

It was several months before I looked at the name on the prescription pad. During that time I tried to convince myself I simply had a good case of empathy with my mother. Even though we'd been a thousand miles apart, I'd had such sharp pain in my breast that it took my breath away, at the very hour of her mastectomy two years before. It seemed logical I would be subject to other psychosomatic symptoms. Finally I made my appointment.

"Mrs. Buchanan, please take a seat and, if you will, fill out these forms for me," the receptionist said, handing me a clipboard and a pen. Filling out forms was near the top of my list of *un*favorite things to do. I could remember the name of every person I'd ever met, but could barely recall my own phone number and address, much less my parents' birthdays and the dates of our various illnesses and surgeries.

Scanning the small print, my eyes jumped to midway on the page. Like a neon sign in a window, the words flashed at me: *Cause of death? Cause of death? Cause of death?* I had to look up to clear my head. Finally, I managed to control my emotions and fill in the spaces: mother's maiden name, birthdate, birthplace, if deceased give *cause of death;* father's name, birthdate, birthplace, living, deceased, if deceased give *cause of death*. The words began flashing again.

Daddy had died of cancer at fifty-two. Mother had been diagnosed with breast cancer and had been given a less than hopeful prognosis. Cause of death? I tried not to think about it.

What I remember about this examination is the small towel. "Strip to the waist and lie down on the table," the nurse instructed as though she'd said it a thousand times before. "Lay the towel across your front," she added, handing me a small rectangle of terry cloth. When the door closed behind her, I did as I was told.

The towel was useless. If it covered one breast, it didn't begin to cover the other. I tried folding it into a triangle, thinking I'd use the old catty-cornered method. It still didn't reach. I tried lying on my side, resting on my elbow with my head propped against my hand. With the other arm, I held the towel in place. It felt like a pose for a sleazy magazine.

When the doctor appeared in the examining room half an hour later, I reminded him we'd been on an Easter Seals telethon together a few years earlier, but he just looked at me as though he didn't have the vaguest idea what I was talking about. He was neither as suave nor as sophisticated as I'd remembered him. He was large, had a bush of unkempt hair, and looked middle-aged (*provided* his life expectancy was one hundred and thirty!).

"Does this hurt? How about this? And this?" he asked as he poked and probed my left breast. It didn't. Then he repeated the procedure on my right breast. When finished, he tried to cover my chest with the postage stamp towel. I gave him no assistance, and it lay between both breasts, covering neither.

I watched as he matter-of-factly made notes on a little yellow scratch pad. "A mammogram . . . you'd better have a mammogram as a precaution," he muttered as he wrote. "I don't *feel* anything or expect to *find* anything, but it never hurts to check it out." He glanced at me and then stepped toward the door.

"Just a minute," I said to his back. He stopped. "My breast *does* hurt. Well, not exactly hurt, but there is an overall discomfort I can't explain."

He turned and smiled. "That's actually a pretty good sign that there's no serious problem." With that, he disappeared.

I don't recall anything about the mammogram or even where I went to have it. I only remember too-small-towel doctor calling a few days later and telling me everything was fine. Before hanging up, he, too, said not to worry.

Idiot! Of course I'll worry, I thought, *I'm out of my mind with worry.*

For the next year I tried to force the thought of cancer from my mind, but the pain in my breast became more than a heaviness. It became very real. I sometimes awakened in the morning with my right hand cupping my left breast, knowing that I had been trying to comfort it even in my sleep.

I remember one such morning in particular. It was the day after I attended the funeral of my friend, Julia, who died of breast cancer. I lay there in bed unable to move because of the honest-to-goodness pain. It was quiet in the house. I turned over on my right side. The sensation was worse without the mattress beneath my breast. I lay on my back; the pain persisted. With a sigh, I rolled back to my left side. My mind began to play "What ifs?" *What if I have cancer? What if I die? What if I leave my children motherless? What if Wayne likes his second wife better than me?*

No pain with breast cancer. If I had a quarter for every time I heard that, from my various doctors and friends who quoted *their* doctors to the interns who examined me in the hospital the night before my surgery, I'd have money for eyeshadow for this life and the next. Mother's doctor had also insisted there is no pain with breast cancer, yet she suffered a gnawing, toothachey pain long before her malignancy was diagnosed.

My fear of cancer grew as the months passed, and my mother's hold on life had become increasingly tenuous. I'd seen my beautiful, life-loving mother grow weaker. Lose hope. Give up. I'd seen her body become emaciated—and, dear God—I was haunted by the vacant stare in her eyes. In those eyes, I began to see my own reflection, and it scared me. *No matter what the doctor says* . . . I thought to myself. Though I still couldn't feel a lump, I decided it was time to go "doctor shopping."

One day when I had a slight cold, I called a physician's listing service and was given the name and phone number of a young doctor, Edmond Tipton, who they told me had recently set up practice and was looking for patients. I made an appointment and decided to put him to the test. "I'm doctor shopping for myself and my family, and here's what I want. I want you to know who we are when we call or visit. I want you to remember our names and something about us. Fake it if you must. I want you to take our phone calls or at least get back to us right away. And I don't want us to wait unreasonable lengths of time to see you." I took in a quick breath, and continued, "In return, we'll pay our bills on time. We'll speak highly of you. And we won't call you unless absolutely necessary—and that includes in the middle of the night. Take it or leave it!"

Grinning broadly, Dr. Tipton stuck out his hand and said, "It's a deal!" He was the only doctor who examined my breast who didn't tell me not to worry. He listened to my story, checked me thoroughly, and admitted he didn't have an answer. "If you listen to your body, it will usually let you know when there's a problem," he said. "And I think we should keep looking until we get an answer. Let's get a specialist to examine you, a surgeon who sees a lot of these cases."

I didn't ask what cases he was referring to, but the words and the fact that I was being referred to a surgeon made my stomach turn.

A few days later when I arrived for my appointment with the surgeon, I was tired of the forms, tired of answering the same questions, tired of the unknown, tired of taking off my bra and tucking it under my blouse. *This is it,* I thought. *There's not a thing wrong with me. Some women go from one doctor to another looking for God-knows-what, and I don't intend to be one of them. When this doctor tells me I have nothing to worry about, I'll never think about it again.*

I sat on the examining table with my feet dangling off the end. Within minutes the doctor entered, before I could even think about turning his pictures upside down.

"What seems to be the problem?" he asked without a hint of a smile. Why couldn't he at least say, "Hello, nice day." *I get a better welcome from the man at the cleaners and spend a fraction of the money,* I thought to myself. I bit my tongue.

As I regurgitated my recent medical history, this new doctor stood with his hands on his hips, like a cowboy. He listened intently, one eyebrow cocked. I told him about the heaviness. The pain. The feeling of foreboding. I had no more to say, but for some reason he intimidated me with his fervent gaze, so I kept right on talking, babbling as if I were stupid.

"Well, you know, my mother has breast cancer. My father died of cancer. And then just recently I went to a funeral in West Virginia for a childhood friend who had breast cancer. I know this other woman who has cancer, and I'm sure it's just all in my head, probably psychosomatic, but then I guess it should be checked out . . ."

"I don't feel any irregularity," he said after I'd finally shut up and he'd examined my breasts, "but you have such large breasts it's hard to tell."

"Try one more thing," I suggested. "Let me show you where to put your hand." The humor didn't escape me. I thought it was probably the first time a naked-to-the-waist woman had to show a man where to put his hand. I sat up and placed his hand on the left and underside of my breast. His hand dug into my flesh as he frowned at the ceiling.

"Well, here again, it's hard to tell. There may be a slight thickening there. How about pain? Is there pain?"

"Yes. Sometimes. Well, almost continually. No! All the time. Yes, all the time," I babbled self-consciously.

"Don't worry. There's no pain with breast cancer," he said rather gruffly. "Unless, of course, it's in the latter stages." My stomach did a flip at that. *Thanks for the comforting words!* I thought.

"I see a lot of women, and I don't think you have cancer. Just to be sure, let's get a mammogram."

"I just had one a few months ago, and it was clear."

"We'll have another, and it'll be a good basis for comparison," he said. Then he turned on his heels and was gone.

As I headed for the parking lot and drove down West End Avenue to have a mammogram, my brain tried to sort out the mixed signals it was receiving: "Nothing to worry about," on one hand; "Unless it's in the latter stages," on the other.

Since my first mammogram, our company, Dynamic Media, had produced several videos for the health care industry. I'd acted as director, so everything was familiar to me. We'd filmed the mammogram process more than once: the waiting room; the forms; the cold, sterile machines; the helpful technicians. I wished for my own cameras and crew, and I wished—oh, how I wished—for an actress to play my role. We'd finish up, and then we'd all go have a cup of coffee. This wasn't a film. This was real life, and the life on the line was mine.

I felt big and bulky next to the slim little technician and wondered why I was always so embarrassed for another woman to see my breasts. I figured she probably saw hundreds a week, but I couldn't help wondering if she went home at night and said to her husband, "I had a patient today with the biggest—or the smallest or the weirdest—breasts I've ever seen!" Probably not. Just routine, all in a day's work.

She touched my shoulder as she guided me toward the big cylinder of a machine and the horizontal, stainless steel surface that would support my breast. "Step as close as you can, open your gown, and place your left breast on the shelf," she said gesturing as if acting out the procedure. When my breast was in place, she adjusted the shelf for my height and pulled another steel plank down, sandwiching my breast between.

"At least you give me something to work with," she laughed. "If you ever want to give some away, I could use it," she added, pointing to her own chest. "It's almost impossible to get my flat-as-two-fried-eggs into position for the procedure." We both laughed. She stepped behind the partition—her protection—and the machine whirred. Before disappearing with the film, she asked me not to dress until the radiologist was sure he had a good picture.

The wait seemed to take longer than it should have, and when she finally returned, it was to report that we needed to repeat the process. "Sometimes, we just get a bad shot," she said. She then took several more exposures.

Again I waited. *They don't know what they're doing,* I told myself, preferring to think they were incompetent rather than to admit something might be wrong with my breast. After what seemed like an eternity, the technician told me I could dress. I'd be called with the report.

The next day was a busy one, so I didn't think once about the mammogram. After all, it was nothing to worry about, just a safeguard, right? I had a client in my office, and we were excitedly reviewing some projects when my secretary buzzed the inner-office phone line. "I normally wouldn't interrupt," she apologized, "but it's your doctor, and he says it's urgent."

I punched the flashing button.

He said his name, and then, "I just talked to the radiologist on your mammogram and it looks like there's a problem."

My mind raced. "What do I need to do?" I asked, careful not to let my client sense my concern.

"Well, we need a biopsy. I wouldn't wait if I were you. When can we arrange it?"

"Tomorrow," I answered numbly and hung up. My client surely must have been puzzled. I hurried him through his appointment. Later I couldn't remember what we had discussed.

When I was finally alone in my office, I sat at my desk, mindlessly shuffling papers. The timing couldn't have been worse. Mother had been admitted to the hospital again, and I had planned to leave immediately for Florida to visit her. What excuse could I give her for not coming? I didn't want to alarm her, but how could I possibly keep my secret from this person with whom I had shared everything. She was the only one in my life who could hold me, rock me, and understand my fear that I too might be dying of cancer.

I didn't know where I had heard it, but the aphorism "Just when you figure out what life's all about, you die!" flashed into my mind, followed by, "The only sure thing in life is death." I'd heard a television preacher say that. And then I remembered how, years before, Aunt Annie would read the obituaries aloud and pronounce to all who would listen: "It'll getcha someday. Sure as shootin', it'll getcha!"

Scenes from the past reeled through my head like motion pictures. When I was little, my cousin Nancy died of spinal meningitis, and they put her in a glass-top casket just like Sleeping Beauty. Until then, I thought just old people died. As I grew, my perspective changed about who was old. Daddy was young when he died at fifty-two; it seemed so unfair that he would never know my children. I wished he could have lived as long as Grandma Nelson, who died at ninety-seven. She fought death tooth and nail, hanging on to her last breath as long as possible.

I was raised in a Christian home and had accepted Christ as my Savior as a young teenager. I had no doubt I would go to heaven and eternal life when I died. I even knew Scripture that said, "To be absent from the body and to be present with the Lord." The dying process was never that much of a mystery to me, but at forty-five I certainly wasn't ready to do it!

Then again, maybe I wouldn't be ready even when I was old. Aunt Lucy, who was old when she died, always said, "The longer you live, the longer you want to live!"

When any of my mother's relatives died, their bodies were brought to the "old home place" in southern Ohio. Located miles from town and the nearest hotel, the house was big enough to accommodate all who wanted to come for the wake, which usually lasted two or three days. Since someone died fairly often in our extended family, I got used to walking through the dimly lit parlor in the middle of the night, past the casket, to the bathroom. As children, my cousins, Nancy, Dianne, and Janice, and I sometimes tried to scare each other by saying we saw the dead person move or by telling horror stories about people waking up six feet underground and trying to claw their way out. I never believed any of that, though. I actually thought of death as a peaceful, natural thing, especially if the person was in heaven, as I'd been taught.

My mind drifted back to Daddy's final days. Even though he had a year of dreadful suffering, his last day on earth was a bright and shining moment in my memory. The sun streamed through the windows of the back bedroom where he lay wracked with pain and weighing less than sixty-five pounds. His last words to me were: "It's so beautiful!" His eyes were shut, and I knew he was seeing something I couldn't see.

I left his room (the one he shared with Mother to the end) and walked to the back door. Even though the sun had been blazing moments before, a light rain was now falling. I gazed out over the backyard which was level for about twenty feet before merging with a steep hillside as many West Virginia yards do. As I stood in the doorway, I saw a beautiful, but mysterious, path of yellow rose petals stretching up the slope as far as I could see. I opened the screen door and stepped out onto the porch. The fragrance of roses was overwhelming. It was something I'll never forget because there were no yellow rose bushes in the yard or the neighbors' yards. I read somewhere that "coincidence is God's way of remaining anonymous." The rose petals, perhaps, were put there by a loving heavenly Father, who cared enough to send the very best.

After a few minutes, I returned to Daddy's room. The sun was once again streaming through the windows. His breathing had stopped. He was gone to investigate what he had glimpsed and pronounced "beautiful" only moments before. As I looked at his still body, a long-forgotten Scripture made its way through the foggy corridors of my mind: "Blessed are the dead who die in the Lord . . . they . . . rest . . ."

Sitting in my office, shuffling papers and thinking of these things, I felt comforted and at peace. Death was not to be feared. But just as I felt that comfort, my mind fast-forwarded to the present. I began thinking about the reality of tomorrow's biopsy, the probability of the diagnosis, and the awful finality of going through the rest of my life without a breast—or worse. Wracked with all of my old fears, I buried my head in my hands, and hot, vulnerable tears filled my eyes. Tomorrow was just a day away!

3

No Mastectomy?!!

I woke early. As I lay in bed, my mind bounced around like one of those balls connected by a rubber band to a wooden paddle. "It's cancer, I know it's cancer, I'll be dead!" *BOING!* (The ball hit the paddle!) "I'll live, I'll live, the biopsy will be benign." *BOING!* (It hit again!) "I won't see my daughters grow to adulthood." *BOING!* "It's cancer, but I'll be brave, I'll be strong, so strong people will think I'm a saint." *BOI-OI-OING!*

The paddle ball dialogue continued as I dressed and drove to the doctor's office—and didn't stop as I sat in the waiting room. After a few minutes I was called into the inner sanctum. The wait there was brief, perhaps because I was the first appointment of the day or maybe, just maybe, he understood the agony I was going through. He spoke very positively.

"I'm just not convinced of a malignancy. It's certainly not clear from the mammogram," he said as once again he examined the breast in question.

"Probably nothing, but if we do get in there and find a problem, we'll need to take the breast." *BOING!* I wanted to pound my head to stop the interference.

"Not at all like we used to do," he continued, ". . . used to do a radical, take *everything*." He began to explain what he meant by everything, but I didn't listen. I knew! With Mother they'd taken everything. Her poor chest looked as though she'd been attacked by a crazed person with an ax. It was concave and discolored; even the movement of her arm was severely impaired. Yes, I knew!

"Today we do what's called a modified radical. It's much less disfiguring," he said as though he expected me to be overjoyed. He explained that along with my breast he would remove and test lymph nodes and if there was "node involvement" (words I would hear often in the future), he would recommend an oncologist to oversee my chemotherapy *BOING!* or radiation *BOING!*

The words were scary to me. Chemotherapy! Radiation! Mother had had both. I didn't want to think about it. After I dressed, he asked me to sign a form giving permission to do a mastectomy if a malignancy was discovered.

"If you were my wife, I'd want that cancer out of there in a hurry." His words made sense, and I signed without a second thought. He patted my shoulder. I left.

With nothing better to do, I drove to Rebecka's Lingerie Shop to buy a new nightie. Rebecka's is the place to go when you want something really special, and I'd had enough "really specials" that Lillian, who waited on me, knew me by name.

"So, Suzanne—the name on my checks—what's the special occasion?" The ball hit the paddle!

Lillian listened as I explained, then she hugged me. "You're a beautiful woman," she said. "I hope you don't have to have a mastectomy, but if you do you'll still be beautiful and Rebecka's carries prostheses and the necessary bras." She seemed pleased to be able to tell me that, as if to say "one less thing to think about."

"Let's not even worry about that right now," she said.

My purchases included an elegant robe and matching gown and a cute little short number that showed off my legs to their best advantage. I bought not one, not two, but three one-of-a-kind satin pillowcases with antique lace out to there.

At around three in the afternoon, Wayne went with me to the hospital. Waiting for me in the admitting office was the most gigantic pot of yellow daffodils you can imagine. So beautiful and so obviously out of season that they were oohed and ahhed over by each passerby. Somehow I knew before I looked at the card that they were from my best friend, Joy.

I filled out the forms, checked into the assigned room, donned my elegant peignoir, and stacked my satin pillows behind my back. Various busy little hospital bees buzzed in to draw blood, take temperature, measure blood pressure, spout questions, and check off lists. One of the practical nurses was a big, beautiful, black woman whom I loved immediately. She knew how to bypass the usual necessities of conversation and get to real talk.

"Oooh, girl . . . look at you! . . . all those fancy pillows. This looks like a house of ill repute!" She twisted the words around her tongue and spat them out like a mouthful of spoiled cottage cheese.

"What're you two gonna do in this room?" she chattered as she worked. "I better shut that door 'fore somebody looks in here."

Some folks came to be helpful, recited their well-rehearsed speeches, and moved on:

* "Hi, I'm your anesthesiologist. Just stopping by to introduce myself and tell you the procedure for tomorrow morning."

* "Excuse me, I'm your dietician with your menu for tomorrow. However, our I-Vs are actually tastier than our food."

* A battle-ax of a nurse marched through the door with nail polish remover and a ball of cotton. "Remove the polish from your fingernails and toenails. I'll be back to check." No excuse me, please, or thank you. I didn't argue with Big Nurse Battle-ax. I removed!

Late in the afternoon my friend Joy came, and Wayne left to go to the office for a while and then bring back some "decent food."

"Joy," I said, "I think I've made a mistake. I shouldn't have signed that paper giving permission for them to do a mastectomy. First of all, I don't want to be put to sleep wondering whether or not I'll wake up without a breast, and secondly, I've read there is a possibility of error—though a remote one—and they could remove my breast unnecessarily."

"Well, go to the nurses' station and get your orders. We'll change them," Joy said with bravado. Joy and I met twenty-five years ago when our husbands were in business together. We were best friends at first sight, and through the years our relationship has only grown stronger. I call her my unofficial publicity person because often when I meet somebody new, they'll say, "Oh, so *you* are Sue Buchanan! I'm so glad to meet you! Joy MacKenzie has told me all about you. She thinks you are wonderful!" Then, of course, I have to try to be wonderful and live up to the person's expectation level. Now that I think of it, it hasn't been easy being Joy's friend!

"Can I do that?" I asked. "Can I change the doctor's orders?"

"Hey, it's your body," she answered. "Of course you can. Probably make your doctor mad, but you can do anything you want to do. You're paying the bills."

"Probably make the doctor mad" was the understatement of the day. I *did* change the orders. Joy went with me to the nurses' station where I asked for my records and a pen.

"NO MASTECTOMY!!!" I wrote across the top of the page and again in the margin next to where I'd signed my permission—three exclamation marks and all—"LUMPECTOMY ONLY!!!"

Perhaps it was because the nurse had given me a wide-point magic marker, but I'll have to admit, the words did have an angry look about them. We went back to the room.

It wasn't five minutes before my surgeon, in his wrinkled scrubs, bolted through the door and assumed his cowboy pose, eyes a-flashin' like a coyote had got his best longhorn. He stared at me and my pillowcases for an inordinately long time before he spoke. In fact it was body language he spoke, and I'd never seen it spoken so fluently! He looked riotously funny—like a big, mad, green frog—and after a few seconds Joy and I burst into laughter. He glared!

Finally he spoke, and though I've forgotten the exact words, basically he told me I was a stupid woman who couldn't face reality, and no matter what my reasons, I shouldn't question his superiority. I tried to explain that I fully intended to have the mastectomy once the reports were in, but before I could get the words out of my mouth he told me in no uncertain terms that having two surgeries was ridiculous when it could all be taken care of in one. His glaring intensified!

As crazy as it may seem, Joy and I were struck with another round of laughter. Joy was literally bent double, holding her stomach, and tears were rolling down my cheeks. It occurred to me it was not the way to treat a person who, in just a few hours, would be standing over me with an assortment of sharp knives.

Disgustedly he threw his hands in the air with a "Hurrumph!" and an I-give-up-and-I-don't-like-it-one-bit gesture and left the room. But not before Joy taunted, "Your clothes are wrinkled too." We both knew he heard and we knew it was rude, but we continued to laugh until we couldn't laugh anymore. This was a turning point for me. Suddenly I was in control and I liked the feeling. I would be making the decisions for my own body from now on.

The evening was a pleasant one. Wayne was there along with my daughter Melinda, who was in high school. Mindy could walk in a room, move a few things around, and suddenly make a blah room look homey and comfortable. She kissed me, smoothed my hair, climbed into bed with me, and leaned back against the gaudy array of pillows.

"I'm staying!" she announced.

My older daughter, Dana, was in college in Indiana and would keep in touch by phone. Friends dropped by, and each person commented on fancy me in my fancy gown in my fancy bed. At nine, everyone left and I didn't feel so very fancy. I dreaded a sleepless night of unanswered questions. Just then there was a rap at the door, and handsome male eyes peered around the corner.

"Carlana told me about you," he said as he came into the

room and turned a chair in my direction. I figured from the clues—a dangling stethoscope and a scrub-cap gollywompased over one eye—he was a doctor of some sort.

"I'm Pat Maxwell," he said as he sat down, stretching his legs halfway across the room. I suspected he'd had a long day.

"Do you know about reconstructive surgery?" he asked.

I was embarrassed to admit that this was one more thing I knew nothing about. The verbiage of the last two days had proved me ignorant of so many things: *lumpectomy* vs. *mastectomy*, *node involvement, chemotherapy, radiation, prosthesis, special bras*. The list was endless.

"No, I don't know a single thing about reconstructive surgery. I've never even heard of it. Tell me."

"Right now, we don't even know if you'll lose your breast," he said. (I would soon find out that Dr. G. Patrick Maxwell was not only Nashville's leading plastic surgeon, but was known throughout the nation as well.)

"If you do, then we'll make you a new one."

"And how do you plan to accomplish that?" I asked. ". . . think you're God or something?"

He quickly and easily picked up on the banter, giving me the impression that yes, if necessary, he did intend to play god in that one area of my life.

"Mind if I take a look?" he said as he pulled aside my gown. "Maybe, in this case I can do a little better job than God," he teased, as he looked at my large beginning-to-sag breasts. His face and tone of voice became serious. "There are different procedures, depending on the circumstances." He stood up and motioned for me to do the same.

"Bend forward," he said and I did as I was told. As I bent he took a handful of my stomach, gave it a little shake and said, "Be glad for this." Then he explained he could rebuild my breast from my stomach fat. That was the craziest thing I'd ever heard. My mind immediately did a good news-bad news joke on me: "The bad news is you might lose your breast. The good news is, you're fat!"

"Let's get the biopsy over. If it's malignant, come see me at my office; I'll talk to you about your options and show you pictures of patients who've had reconstructive surgery. I'll try to give you all the information you'll need to make a wise decision." He wished me luck and said goodnight. The mild sedative I'd taken earlier had begun to relax me, and soon drowsiness was overtaken by a deep, deep sleep.

In another part of the hospital my brother and sister-in-law checked in to have their very first baby. They'd waited a long time for this moment; not only the usual nine months, but before that, a lengthy time of doubt and testing, wondering whether or not they could conceive.

The next morning I was kept groggy until time to be wheeled to surgery. Wayne came early, and my brother stopped by to give me a progress report from the maternity ward. He told me that Becky was tired after such a long labor, but that everything was okay. "I've eaten every bag of peanut M&Ms in the vending machine," he added.

Joy was there to keep Wayne company. If anyone could buoy his spirits, it was she.

A nurse came to give me another needleful of groggy. I had a hard time staying awake. I had no worries. Finally the gurney pushers came. I kissed my husband, gave my friend a hug, and was whisked away and put soundly to sleep.

I knew nothing, of course, about what happened next. I often wondered how soon Wayne knew the results and who told him the bad news. If it was the doctor, I wondered what he said. Recently, I asked my husband to fill in the gaps.

"Want to read my journal?" he asked.

"What journal?" Imagine my surprise when he pulled a big red notebook off the shelf. He thumbed the pages till he found the right place.

"Read!" he said.

From where I was sitting, I could see him coming down the long hall. There were two nurses with him, one on either side. He was dressed in "operating room green," and the scrub cap was pushed back on his head. He still had on the cloth shoe coverings that caused him to sort of shuffle as he walked.

Jon, Sue's younger brother, was sitting across the bed opposite Joy and me. He was beaming from ear to ear. After all, that's what men are supposed to do when they've just been presented with a magnificent baby girl (the first one) less than an hour earlier. He had never known such unrestrained excitement and justifiable pride.

Joy leaned over to me and nodded toward the hallway as if to say: "That's he, isn't it?" She didn't ask the question out loud; she knew I'd already seen the surgeon coming. My eyes were glued on him, and my whole body was tense, even though I like to pride myself in always appearing to be totally in control.

He came in and stood beside Jon even though he didn't acknowledge Jon's or Joy's presence. He was obviously in a hurry and wasn't there to exchange pleasantries or small talk. He looked and spoke directly to me, using as few words as necessary to consummate his mission.

"We completed the procedure and the preliminary lab tests show that the tumor is malignant—about the size of a lead pencil eraser." He held his hand out, pointing with his thumb to the tip of his little finger.

"Quite small," he said. "The final lab work will be completed later today and I'll know more about the type of cancer it is after I review the results of the culture from pathology. Then we'll discuss the next steps. Your wife is doing quite nicely; she's in recovery and should be back to the room in a little while. Any questions?"

That was like asking a drowning man if he'd like someone to throw him a rope—of course he would, but with a mouth full of water, how can he answer? My mouth was totally dry, glued shut with emotion; my mind was bland; my body was limp and I felt numb. All I could manage to do was shake my head from side to side. Anguish rushed in to consume the optimism and hope that had been there just seconds before.

Jon broke down, sobbing uncontrollably. He'd been from the height of ecstasy to the depth of despair in less than two minutes. In that same hospital, on the very same day, within the span of an hour, his wife had given birth to their child—a little girl—and he got the news his sister had cancer. I sat there too stunned, too overwhelmed with my own grief to move, to help my best friend, my brother-in-law. Joy, who had come to comfort, simply tightened her lips, touched my arm, then looked tearfully away, fully realizing there were no words appropriate for the moment.

By the time I came back to the room from surgery, Wayne had managed to pull himself together. No matter what Wayne felt inside, I saw a smiling face and heard encouraging words. Other than a bandage on my chest I looked and felt the same. When I asked the question, "Was it malignant?" my husband answered that it was and repeated the doctor's words as to the size of the tumor, emphasizing "small as a pencil eraser."

Human nature somehow allows us to adjust information to make it possible to digest. I adjusted the information emphasizing the word *small* as I repeated it in my head. With a big grin Wayne changed the subject.

"You have a new niece," he said, and for the time being we were able to turn our thoughts to that happy event. He told me her size and weight and reported that Becky was doing fine. We discussed possible names, and I wondered if anyone had told Mother or if she was too sick to understand she had a new grandchild.

Later that afternoon Jon and Becky came to my hospital room and placed a tiny pink bundle in my arms.

"Cara Jane Davis, meet your Aunt Sue," my brother said.

I've loved Cara ever since that moment. Thirteen months later her sister, Kirby, arrived. Conception was easier the second time around! Redheaded, giggly, energetic Kirby! Her mother lives in total fear of what her next words might be! Cara is a lady, with a face like porcelain, heavy eyebrows, and eyes so expressive they practically speak, which is a good thing, since it's almost impossible to get a word in edgewise with her sister around.

Each time I see Kirby, she takes a running leap at me, kisses me hard on the mouth, and answers, "Fine" before I can say, "How are you?" Cara watches with those beautiful brown eyes, waits till Kirby finishes her song and dance, and then moves close for a hug.

That day in the hospital, holding that less-than-twenty-four-hour life in my arms gave me hope and purpose for living. *They need me,* I thought and remembered Mother saying my brother Joe was born when her mother died and my brother Jon was born when her father died. Then she commented it was "Just like the Bible says—'The Lord giveth and the Lord taketh away.'"

The Lord is giving us Cara and taking away my mother, I thought. And since Mother wouldn't be around to love Jon and Becky's children, it was all the more important for me to be there.

Chapter *4*

The Wonders
of Pink
Play-Doh

A few years ago a powerful publisher was asked if she had ever turned down a book that made her want to bang her head against the wall just thinking about it. She answered that, in fact, she had turned down such a book. The title of it was *I'm OK, You're OK*, which was picked up by another publisher and became a runaway bestseller. When asked why she rejected the book, she answered, probably with a grimace: "Because I was OK!"

I understand that. Before I had cancer, I was okay and had been all my life! Why should anyone *not* be okay, either in mind or body? I suppose, to some extent, I thought health was something I could control with my mind. My parents taught positive thinking right along with Christianity. Instead of "Cleanliness is next to godliness," at our house it was, "Positive thinking is next to godliness!" Like my own parents, I had easy answers for my children.

"Snap out of it!" I'd say, "Stop mullygrubbing!"

God certainly didn't want you to mullygrub. I could think of a dozen verses from the Bible that said "Don't mullygrub." Not in those exact words, of course, but the message was there, not only for living, but for dying as well. In Psalms I knew God promised:

Yea, though I walk through the valley of the shadow of death,
I will fear no evil;
For You are with me;
Your rod and Your staff, they comfort me.

Daddy was a person who trusted that concept completely. He never complained, even though he suffered pain from the ravages of cancer almost every moment for over a year. Theoretically, at least, I knew that when God decided it was my turn to die—bite the bullet, meet my maker, walk into the sunset, shake hands with Elvis—I could exit, drawing from the same source of comfort as my father.

Even though I knew I had a malignancy and would lose a breast, this ingrained bent toward positive thinking drove me like a Mack truck for the next two days. I didn't mullygrub once, and I was in a constant state of *snap-out-of-it-ness!*

The night I came home from the hospital after the biopsy, Wayne and I mapped out a plan. We outlined the next two days and listed every person we knew who could give us information.

See: Dr. Maxwell: body work!
Dr. "Cowboy": surgery and to recommend an oncologist
Oncologist: treatment
2nd oncologist: 2nd opinion
American Cancer Society: literature and information
Lillian: prosthesis and bras

Phone:
Doctor (shirttail relative) in Denver
Doctor (friend of friend) in Tulsa
Various witch doctors (friends of friends) who use unorthodox methods
All the people we know who recovered from cancer to ask them how they did it

The next morning I hit the road running. First to the plastic surgeon, Dr. Maxwell. Visiting his office was like visiting close friends. I'm not sure I understood what it was that first day, but eventually I figured it out. Plastic surgery is in most cases elective (not like having to have your gallbladder out). These people understand marketing and that good clients (patients) beget good clients.

As I walked through the door, my eyes took in the beautiful waiting room. The furniture was arranged in conversation-friendly groupings, unlike the predictable chair-chair-chair-table-chair-chair of most doctors' offices. Not a duck or six-month-old *Newsweek* in sight, but rather various *objets d'art* and big collector books. The receptionist stood up and came toward me.

"We've been waiting for you. I'm Rosemary. Are you doing okay?" she said, and she offered to share her banana bread. "Our patients bring us goodies all the time. I'm getting fat; look at this." She patted her perfect hips. My eyes took in her perfect face.

Of course, I wondered if she had partaken of the glories of plastic surgery, and yes, dear friend, I looked closely at each woman who came into the waiting room, and yes, I played the same guessing game: "Wonder what she's having done . . ." and "Wonder what she's had done . . ." and on and on. I played it that day and every visit after!

It seemed that everyone in the office was just waiting to meet me, to answer my questions, to help me in my crisis. The first thing the doctor did was show me a scrapbook. The pictures there were unbelievable. On the first page there were three pictures, obviously all of the same person even though the face wasn't visible.

My eyes barely glanced at the middle-aged sagging breasts of the first picture. Instead they were drawn like a magnet to picture number two: a maimed torso, minus one breast. In its place was a vicious, ugly scar. The remaining breast stared at me like some eye, some cyclops freak of nature. I sucked in my breath, and my eyes were glued to the atrocity. Dr. Maxwell didn't try to use words to soften the blow. He waited until my eyes moved on to the next photograph.

"What's this?" I asked in awe. "A reconstruction job?" The doctor simply nodded his head in affirmation and I leaned close for a better look at this work of perfection. Two matching, pert, compact breasts, good enough for the cutest little cheerleader I'd ever met!

We continued through the book until I saw breasts very much like my own. I stopped and stared. Big, white, weighty breasts. Obviously the before shots. In the next picture one of those breasts was missing. I couldn't look! I'd seen all I wanted to see of mutilated chests. The third was the after picture. Sure enough, better than they were to begin with. No bag, no sag!

"I understand now why you were so smug the other night. You do give God some competition, don't you?"

He gave me a knowing look and chuckled. I couldn't help remembering a joke I'd heard: It seems there was a lawyer at the gate of heaven who saw a doctor walk past everyone in line, nod to Saint Peter, and walk right in. The lawyer, wanting justice, complained to Saint Peter.

"Who does that doctor think he is, going to the front of the line and walking right in?" "That's not a doctor," Saint Peter replied. "That's God. Sometimes he likes to play doctor."

Pat (Dr. Maxwell didn't seem to mind that somewhere along the way I dropped the formalities of his title) gave me all the time I needed. He drew diagrams in the air as he told me my options and described the various procedures. It was even possible to use a flap from my back and twist it around to the front and insert an implant. He showed me different kinds of implants and discussed the pros and cons of each. I held one and played it from hand to hand like a Slinky toy. I knew about implants; some of my best friends had them, not because of cancer, but for aesthetic reasons.

He explained, in greater detail than he had at the hospital, how he could use my own body tissue—stomach fat and muscle—to rebuild the breast. He'd already *approved* my tummy fat.

"If you do it that way, you get a tummy-tuck in the bargain," he reminded me. What woman in her right mind couldn't see the advantage in that?

That first night Pat had visited me in the hospital, I had wondered about the nipple, whether it could somehow remain intact.

Now I thought, *Of course not. The nipple will be gone, but a reconstructed breast with no nipple is better than no breast at all!*

"Did I explain the nipple?" Pat asked, as if reading my mind.

I shook my head. "In some cases we graft it to another area of the body for the duration of treatment and reposition it at the time of reconstructive surgery. We don't do it, though, when cancer cells are present because of the possibility of spreading the cancer. In your case we'll just make you a new nipple."

"The god syndrome?" I questioned, trying to pretend I wasn't overwhelmed by this new piece of information. "How do you manage that? Pink Play-Doh?"

He laughed and explained that recreating the nipple was the simplest part of the job. He would remove a small portion of skin from the inside of the top of my leg and sew it to the proper place to make the areola. With a few extra stitches he would create a sack that simulates (in looks only) a nipple. He explained that the skin pigment from that part of the leg actually resembles the normal brownish-pink areola color.

"If you have good insurance, it'll most likely pay," he commented. "The only negative thing is that we'll have to wait until after chemotherapy."

This has changed in the years since my surgery, and in most cases today the procedure is done immediately, sometimes in two steps, using an expander to stretch the skin and later replacing it with a permanent implant. He suggested that even though reconstructive surgery was off in the future, he would come to the hospital the morning of my mastectomy and draw lines on my body to show my surgeon where to cut. He explained that often surgeons didn't take his needs into consideration—didn't leave him enough skin to work with—and that if care wasn't taken the scar might be visible above the dress line. Since my cleavage was much like that of the Queen Mother, I'd never worn very low-necked dresses, but I decided to take his word for it.

"One last detail . . ." Dr. Maxwell said as he closed my chart. "Let's get some pictures." We moved to another room, and his assistant, Babs, helped him adjust the lighting. We chatted like old friends, and when I left, I had the feeling they hated to see me go.

My next stop was the surgeon's office, and I felt much less brave than I had in the hospital with my friend Joy present. In fact, as I sat in the waiting room I found myself rehearsing what I'd say when I came face to face with this doctor we'd so blatantly poked fun at. Maybe I'd just throw my arm around his shoulder and say, "Shoot, doctor, I don't know what got into me. I guess you just bring out the worst in me." Or I could blame Joy: "*She* brings out the worst in me and I've told her good-bye, so long, you're a bad influence!" I would promise never to see her again. Maybe I'd mention I'd met Johnny Cash. I'd heard he was Johnny's doctor. Couldn't hurt!

Before I decided which tactic to use, the door opened and the nurse read from my chart: "Mrs. Buchanan!" I could tell from her voice that word had gotten around that I was a troublemaker.

Our company had produced medical videos and one of the subjects was "risk management," which told the doctor how to manage his practice in a way that would help him avoid malpractice lawsuits. One important point was to keep good records. In our research we uncovered the fact that sometimes a doctor writes nasty little acronyms on a patient's chart. We found such things as "RFM," which stands for "Ready for Morgue," and HSLT, for "High Speed Lead Therapy"—or more specifically "shoot the patient!" A pediatrician scribbled UKD, meaning Ugly Kid Disease, and another physician wrote in the space marked prescribed therapy: "Hold pillow to face for four hours—repeat every fifteen minutes." Once we were shooting a video in a Houston hospital, and I personally saw a doctor write, "Sweet Potato Poisoning," on a black man's records.

I couldn't see what my chart said—HSLT most likely—but the doctor's body language flashed the word *condescending* in neon! He was just too, too nice as he checked the incision, repeated the information he'd given me at the hospital, and told me he had arranged for the mastectomy and would see me at the hospital the next day.

"Smaller than a pencil eraser" still had a nice ring to it, even spoken in condescending-ese! He offered, condescendingly, the name of an oncologist in his same building and condescendingly asked if I'd like his "girl" to arrange an appointment. I answered that I would. With something resembling a flair, he took my hand and helped me down from the examination table. He was so nice, I hated to leave!

I was told I could see the oncologist immediately. I took the elevator down two floors, turned the corner, and entered the first door on the left just as I'd been instructed. The office staff seemed cold as Popsicles in the Antarctic, but Dr. Sidney Solomon seemed like a nice guy and a good photographer. Being a photographer myself, I could relate. His studies in black and white were displayed on the walls: cows, barns, old bridges, and junkyard scenes. The same things caught my eye when I went out for the day with my camera.

This doctor had the greatest, most direct, look-you-in-the-eye handshake in the Western world and was receptive to my, "Hey, I'm a photographer too." At least I thought I saw a glimmer in his eye that said he'd remember me if, by some far-out chance, I needed his services. Maybe homemade cookies would warm up the office staff.

I handed him the file folder sent from the surgeon and he opened it. Lymph involvement seemed to be the key factor in determining whether I would need his services. He explained, as had the surgeon, that during surgery, lymph nodes would be removed from under my arm and sent to the lab for testing.

If there were no malignant nodes, there would be no chemotherapy. If there *was* node involvement, the intensity and length of the treatment would depend on how many nodes were positive.

"Three months, six months at the most," he said. I liked him and I liked his photography, so I decided against a second opinion.

I went to my office and tied up loose ends with Abby, my secretary, and on the way home, I stopped at the American Cancer Society to pick up some brochures and books. Then I went home to spend the evening educating myself and making phone calls. Wayne and I talked to a lot of friendly, helpful people that night, but it's a blur now. Nothing changed the fact that the next day I would check into the hospital again and have my breast cut off.

That night Wayne held me close for a long time, and then we made love slowly—deliberately at first—and then so passionately I forgot what lay ahead. I fell asleep, wondering if the same intimacy could ever again be achieved. Someone sobbed silently in the night. It must've been me, aware but not fully awake.

The next morning, in a mad frenzy, I bathed, shaved my legs, removed my nail polish for the benefit of Nurse Battleax, plucked my eyebrows, did laundry, cleaned out the refrigerator, grocery shopped, and went to the beauty shop. Then I called my secretary and went over the list I'd made while I was under the dryer.

Next I headed to Rebecka's where Lillian showed me the various prostheses and bra selections and suggested I come back after my scar healed. At that time she would work with me to find the best choices. While I was there I bought three more gowns and two more pillowcases. I didn't need more pillowcases, but when I commented on how much I liked the ones I'd bought, one thing led to another: Lillian mentioned they were made by a very old lady and—actually it came to us both at once—this could be my last chance to buy more!

Late afternoon I checked into the hospital for the second time in a week. Friends filled the room for the entire evening, laughing, joking, and telling "remember the time" stories. I'm sure the nursing staff, as well as nearby patients, were glad when visiting hours were over. After my friends were gone, Wayne, Mindy, and Dana, who had come home from college, stayed behind. There were tears in our eyes as we kissed goodnight.

A needleful of groggy in my hip made sleep come quickly. The next morning Dr. Maxwell was my first visitor. With a thick, black marker he drew a football shape on my left breast with one end of the football pointed into my armpit, the other toward the opposite hip. The "football" was bottom heavy and encompassed the nipple. He made markings around the nipple.

By the time my family arrived the I-Vs—with groggy added—were in place. I didn't give a rat's ankle what they removed: my breast, my leg, or even my head. The gurney pushers had to pick me up like a rag doll and put me on the cart. Just before they wheeled me away, the phone rang.

"For you," Wayne said and put the phone to my ear.

I recognized the voice of our close friend Doug. Doug and Laura Lee, friends of long standing, had recently moved from Nashville to Ohio. Even though my response was feeble, I was glad to hear his voice.

"Can I pray for you?" he asked.

"Yeah, hurry, I gotta go," I muttered. I'll always remember that sweet prayer holding me up to the heavenly Father and reminding me, as I was on the verge of slipping out of conscious thought, that I was His child, that I was in His hands. I was ready to be wheeled into the operating room.

The first thing I remember when I awoke from surgery was a hallucinogenic-shaped woman hovering over me, repeating, "Suzanne! Suzanne! Do you know where you are? Suzanne! Suzanne! Are you awake? Suzanne! Suzanne! Do you know where you are?"

I was confused. Mother always called me Suzanne when she was angry, but this gossamer lady didn't appear to be angry. Her only intent seemed to be to pull me out of the long, dark anesthetic tunnel that felt so safe into acknowledged pain and the harsh lights of the recovery room. "Suzanne! Suzanne! You're in recovery." She stuck a thermometer in my mouth.

The day was a blur but by evening, except for the six-inch-thick bandage and the knot in my stomach, I felt better. At least the anesthetic was wearing off. Dana insisted on spending the night in the room, and every time I awakened, she was there, rubbing my arm, stroking my hair, asking how I felt. Dana later told me she had been trying to make up for being "rotten" (her word) to me over the past couple of years. She said that during the long night she kept wondering if she perhaps *gave* me cancer.

By morning I'd regained the will to live! Dana helped me adjust the bed so I could look in the mirror. I expected to see Dracula's mother, but to my surprise, my cheeks were pink and my eyes bright. I patted my hair in place with my one good arm, poked around in the drawer for my makeup, and dabbed it in the proper places. I felt good and looked good if you didn't take into account the thick bandage around my chest under the yucky hospital gown.

I never felt really bad again after that first day. A pain here and a pain there, but mostly I felt numb in the area where the breast had been removed. Women often ask me what to expect in the way of pain, both for a mastectomy and reconstructive surgery.

"Think of the surgery as being done on the *surface* of your body," I say, ". . . rather than in your guts." That simplification helped me play down the pain and think of it as "no big deal." What I wasn't prepared for was the emotional pain of losing a breast and the bad prognosis.

Each post-surgery report was worse than the last. At first, the surgeon told us there were nodes involved; next he said "a number of nodes" were involved; and finally, he said that there were fourteen malignant nodes. The oncologist said six months of chemotherapy, then changed it to nine. Finally his words were, "A year of aggressive chemotherapy." A day or so after my mastectomy, the nursing school director came to visit, along with several young student nurses.

"Do you mind if the girls drop in to visit with you?" she asked. "In class they're learning how to relate to a patient and this would help them apply what they learn." Of course, I welcomed the chance to advance the cause of medicine in my own humble little way.

One of the student nurses gave me her undivided attention, practically never leaving my side. She fluffed my pillows, stooped to help me with my slippers, opened my mail, and hovered in the background when visitors were present. She even came by after work. I thought perhaps she was just curious about me—this patient with frou-frou robes and bed jackets, satin pillows with lace out to there, and friends who climbed right into bed with her. One day it slipped out, and I think she had no idea of what she said. She told me she was observing me, a patient facing death!

At about the same time, Dana had returned to college and was sharing her feelings with a friend, a doctor's daughter. After Dana poured out her fears and dreads to this girl, thinking that of all people she would understand, the girl looked at her and calmly said, "Your mother's as good as dead. You may as well get used to it."

The outlook wasn't great, but then again, you *did* hear about people who beat the odds!

I'll be one of those people, I thought to myself. *I'll do whatever it takes. I'll offer up my veins to those rubber-soled women in white! I'll swallow their pills! I'll drink toad spit if necessary! I may complain, but I'll do it!*

Chapter 5

Chemotherapy and My Cat, Ya

When I think about chemotherapy, I think of my cat, Ya, my friend and companion during those dreary months.

I have been owned by many cats in my lifetime, some whose names I've forgotten. Some I named childish names like Baddie and Goodie because they were bad and good; and in fact I was a child. At a very young age, as Mrs. Vandertweezers, I strolled the block with my cat, "Smokey, the Pirate, Don Derk of Don Day," both of us dressed to the nines! For days at a time I wouldn't answer to Sue, only to Mrs. Vandertweezers. Mrs. Vandertweezers, elegant lady that she was, felt her wardrobe rivaled that of any Hollywood star or that of the Queen of England.

Her regal companion, Smokey, the Pirate, Don Derk of Don Day, rode on his back in the baby buggy, dressed in a doll dress and bonnet as Mrs. V strolled past Mrs. Eubanks' house, past the Liebles', past the convent, and past the Catholic school to Sacred Heart Catholic Church and back again.

"Hello, Dahling!" she said to everyone.

"Everyone" was mostly the sisters walking back and forth between church, school, and convent. Sometimes Mrs. Vandertweezers and Smokey, the Pirate, were invited into the convent for a visit and some ice cream. Once they actually made a little turn through the foyer of the church, but they left hurriedly when Father Cuthbert came toward them, his robes flying and his eye on Smokey, the Pirate, Don Derk of Don Day.

Going to that magnificent church and having a string of those nice tiny black beads, doing the little curtsy and being slightly mysterious, was more than a little appealing to Mrs. Vandertweezers, and she gave Catholicism strong consideration. Naturally, she couldn't possibly become a nun because then she couldn't be *Mrs.* Vandertweezers and enjoy her lavish wardrobe.

Then there was Agamemnon, who was the smartest cat ever to own me. He got his name from *The Four Little Kittens,* a book I still have, after all these years. The book begins: "Once upon a time, there were four little kittens. Their names were Buzz, Fuzz, Suzz and Agamemnon." It ends: ". . . when their Mother tucked Agamemnon into bed, she remembered he was the youngest and had tried the hardest. So she gave him an extra kiss on the tip of his nose."

My mother never let me kiss Agamemnon and my other cats on the nose or anywhere else. She said I would get a horrible disease. Now that I have had a horrible disease, I kiss my cats and wonder what Mother would think if she knew.

Among other manifestations of intelligence, Agamemnon could turn the piano light on and off. He would use his claws to grip the pull-chain. On and off it would go, a wonderful distraction when I was supposed to be practicing.

I still have the newspaper clipping that tells of Agamemnon's disappearance and my letter to the Great Scott, our local radio personality, telling him my "best friend" was lost and would he please help find him. I didn't mention that my "best friend" was a cat until the very last line.

Great Scott read my letter over the air, and sure enough, a listener heard my plea and discovered the "guest" in his home was not just an ordinary stray. He should have known! Strays don't stretch out over half the length of the buffet without touching a single piece of crystal. Strays don't sit by the refrigerator, looking at it through half-closed eyes, and then look at you in the same manner, back and forth until you say, "Okay, okay, I'll feed you!" *and* strays do not turn lights on and off! The man brought Agamemnon home, and he lived happily with us for many years.

We think of our cat Ya every year at Christmas when I pull the Christmas tree skirt out of the box and admire its beauty. It wasn't easy, gluing on all those pieces of felt and tiny little sequins. Ladies dancing! Calling birds! French hens! Right over there by the swans a-swimming is a faded brown spot. We look at it each year and say, "Oh, that's where Ya threw up, God rest his soul!" and a tear comes to the eye.

We got Ya when the girls were little. He made the move with us to Nashville and grew old and bored (not bored because of Nashville . . . he just did!). His only claim to fame was that he was true to a comment of Theophile Gautier: "He loved books, and when he found one open on the table he would lie down on it, turn over the edges of the leaves with his paw; and after a while, fall asleep, for all the world as if he had been reading a fashionable novel."

Each week, Wayne and I read the Sunday newspaper, and as we finished with the various parts, we tossed them to the floor and waited. Sure enough Ya would walk around on each section, sometimes stopping on the funnies or the want ads to take a bath, and then curl up on the "Sunday Showcase" for a long afternoon nap. Always the *Sunday Showcase!* That is until I was executive of the week in the "Business Perspective."

That day he skipped the funnies and the want ads, did not glance at sports, fashions, or showcase. He went straight to the "Business Perspective," looked at my picture, read the article, and then chose that exact place to take his nap. We even snapped pictures to prove it!

I hate to say this out loud, but Ya *loved* cancer and *loved* chemotherapy. He was happiest during my year of bad fortune, and he made my life more bearable.

Treatment began five days after my mastectomy, while I was still in the hospital. I've come to believe that beginning so quickly was an incredibly wise decision on the part of my oncologist. "Begin now!" he said. "Remember those cells are reproducing themselves at a staggering rate. We need to catch them before they get a head start on us."

Often a cancer patient tells me her doctor has said there's no hurry to begin treatment. "Get through Christmas . . . or vacation . . . or what have you," he'll say. It seems to me that the longer you wait, the more time you have to dread it. For me, the sooner the better.

The program he set up for me was pretty standard at the time. It called for bombarding my body with chemicals for two weeks and then allowing it to revitalize for two weeks. The bad news was that the drugs destroyed not only the cancer cells but the healthy ones as well. The good news was that the noncancerous cells replenished themselves at a faster speed than the others.

To begin my program each month, I went to Dr. Solomon's office where I was given my initial dose of medicine. On one of my first visits, the scene was so gloomy I wanted to run away. There were three or four women in very bad wigs and one in a turban. A man nodded to me and spoke, and I recognized him as one of Nashville's most powerful lawyers. He was gently helping his elderly father, who was very sick. So much for powerful! Even the rich and influential could not bypass all this.

The patients appeared to have one thing in common: Their complexions had a putrid greenish cast. How soon would I be wearing a wig because of hair loss? How soon would I become bald and green? The waiting time in the reception area seemed endless, yet the hands of my watch had barely moved.

My name was called, and I moved to an inner room, lined with schoolroom-style chairs, the kind with a paddlelike arm on one side. In this case, the extension wasn't a surface for writing notes and assignments but support for my arm which would be elastic-banded so its veins would pop out, then swabbed, needled, and Band-Aided. Sometimes patted!

I had no fear of needles, but I dreaded the process of locating a suitable vein, since mine are exceptionally small. Slap the arm, try for the vein. Slap the arm, try for the vein.

Sometimes the nurse never found the one she was looking for—on the inside of my arm at the elbow—and had to use the one on the back of my hand where it caused ugly bruising and was a constant reminder of the painful procedure. I had a favorite nurse named Pat, who could find the vein on the first try. I prayed each time that she would be available.

Once the needle was in my arm, various cylindrical vials could be attached without having to insert a new needle each time. First the nurse attached an empty vial to the shaft drawing blood that she immediately handed to a technician who tested it for the telltale signs of cancer. Next, one by one, slowly and meticulously the two medications were administered.

Next I went into an examination room, pulled off my clothes from the waist up, put on the sleeveless paper top as instructed, and literally held my breath, waiting to know the outcome of the blood test. I rarely had to wait long. Before the doctor even shut the door behind him, he told me what I wanted to know: "The bloodwork looks fine!" I appreciated the fact he didn't make me wait. I wonder if I ever thanked him.

"Let's take a look," he'd say as he poked around checking my chest, neck, and abdomen for lumps or swelling that might indicate a problem. Next he looked in my mouth and down my throat checking for mouth sores. On the days when my blood count was low, sure enough, my mouth was full of sores. Those times he usually postponed the treatment. Besides conversation about my health, we chatted. I was traveling back and forth to New York City on business at the time. He had been raised and educated there and loved recommending restaurants and jazz clubs to me. I returned the favor by suggesting local restaurants to him. He'd been out of circulation, busy doing doctor things, and had no idea where to go in Nashville for a romantic evening. I introduced him and his fiancé to a quaint little restaurant in Clarksville an hour or so away. It was important to me to establish some sort of relationship with this person, who was perhaps my link to life itself. I liked him and I knew he liked me.

As we talked, he wrote out my prescription for two weeks of pills, part of the total protocol, plus something for nausea, if I needed it. (I always did!) A week later I returned for my second bombardment of the month and, except for the prescription, repeated the process. Every other month I had a chest X-ray.

Because of everything I'd heard about chemotherapy, I had a mind-set against it from the beginning. I *expected* it to make me sick. The doctor's office smelled like a chemical factory, and the aftertaste in my mouth was how I imagined dry cleaning fluid would taste. Right from the beginning, I fussed and stewed about this yucky stuff. In my mind, I called it every bad name I could think of. I regarded the visits to the doctor's office a nuisance. "A ridiculous waste" was my label for the time I had to reserve for recuperation after treatment. It was ridiculous that I had to put up with this interference in my busy schedule.

After a couple of months of fighting against everything chemotherapy represented, I had a life-shaking experience. One day as I waited for the doctor to come through the door with his pronouncement, I couldn't sit still. I began to beat my fists against the padded examining table, mumbling the four letter word I'd ascribed to chemotherapy. "——, ——, ——, it's nothing but——!" I said. The word describes it well, I thought to myself.

Call me a skeptic, but before that day, had someone told me that he or she had personally heard the audible voice of God, I would've called for the padded wagon!

It wasn't weird or strange, and it may not have been audible, but it was real. It was gentle and familiar, and it simply said, "Don't fight. This is good. It's from Me. Accept this medicine into your body and let it work for you and make you well. Thank Me for it. Thank Me!"

I believe I may have answered. "Okay, Lord!" I'm not sure, but I do know that from that day forward, I didn't mullygrub about chemotherapy. I waltzed into that little room, pulled off my clothes, put on the sticky little bolero, raised my hands to God, and thanked Him. I even elaborated on His directions. "Take the medicine and put it where it will do the most good . . ." I'd say as I ran my hands over my body, ". . . and thank You, God. Thank You from the bottom of my heart!"

Later, at home, I began to spend more time thanking God, not only for the medicine and the medical professionals, but for my husband who enjoyed making my life easy, my daughters who loved me dearly, and my friends who supported me in every way. One of those friends gave me a colorful book called *The Human Body,* a children's book, and I began incorporating the illustrations into my prayers.

"This is a picture of a healthy brain, Lord. Help mine to be healthy and free from cancer." I did the same with the pictures of liver, lungs, and bones, the likely places breast cancer would metastasize. The pictures certainly didn't help God. He knew what my guts looked like. It helped me.

The first two or three months chemotherapy made me tired, and I went home and slept the afternoon away after treatment. I felt progressively worse each month, eventually throwing up at the thought of the procedure.

Each time I went for chemo, Wayne took me and picked me up. He offered to go in with me, but I knew he needed to be at the office, and I knew sometimes a doctor tends to "talk around" a patient when a spouse is present. Instead, I wanted a strong partnership between my doctor and me.

My appointment was at one o'clock in the afternoon, allowing me a productive morning in the office. Afterward Wayne took me home and turned me over to Ya for the afternoon. Ya would curl into the curve of my body and we would both sleep the afternoon away. The nausea became progressively worse each month. It hit late in the afternoon, and I was sick—so sick—through the evening and into the night. Ya was tolerant. When I was in the bathroom, he took the opportunity to have his evening meal and his bath, but each time I returned to bed, he was waiting to cuddle and comfort.

On the day of my treatment, I must have looked and felt worse than my childhood cat Agamemnon did after he'd been out for two or three days and nights at a time, doing whatever it is tomcats do! He used to drag his big, old, yellow body through the door, turn his ears back at the food we offered, flop down, and with all the energy he could muster, lick his wounds—sometimes bloody, once with part of an ear missing—and give us a look that said, "Do not disturb!" Then he'd sleep the day away.

On the day after my treatment, I'd drag myself out of bed, turn my nose up at food (the people version of cats turning their ears back), and lick my wounds. The nausea came now and then, but lessened as the day progressed. Eventually, I'd try a piece of toast with a tiny bit of peanut butter. Dear friends, Ronn and Donna Huff, sent a fruit or juice basket each time I had a treatment and I came to look forward to the goodies tucked inside. By evening I'd comb my hair, put on lipstick, and welcome my husband. By the third day I was back at work behaving like a normal person.

One of the worst things a chemotherapy patient has to deal with is loss of hair. I hated sitting in the doctor's waiting room with other cancer patients who were in that predicament. Women wore their turbans and wigs. Men sometimes wore ball caps, but more likely than not, they wore nothing on their heads at all, their bald heads shining like chrome on a Cadillac.

"Your hair usually falls out around the seventh week," I was told. Knowing that it would happen was bad enough. Knowing the timing of when it would happen gave me a permanent knot in the pit of my stomach. It occurred to me that being prepared might help. I would buy my wig ahead of time. Once I discovered that my insurance would pay for it, I decided to have one handmade, not only to match the *color* of my hair, but the style as well. Someone recommended a beautician, a wig specialist and former cancer patient herself.

My new wig was a perfect match, but it didn't ease the knot in my stomach. I was told that someday I'd wake up and my hair would be on my pillow . . . or in the bottom of the shampoo bowl. I wished it would happen and be over with.

Mary Edith, a friend from church, came to my house and prayed for me: "Lord, please don't let Sue lose *all* her hair." The Lord chose to answer that prayer, exactly as it was prayed! I didn't lose *all* my hair. Just about two-thirds of it. Fortunately, because it was quite long at the time, it could be wound around my head to camouflage the bald spots. Through the years I've wondered why the Lord did it the way He did. At first I thought it must be some sort of divine joke. It seems to me, if the God of the universe was going to get involved in my dilemma at all, He would do it up big and see to it I didn't lose one single little hair. I've come to the conclusion that perhaps He let me lose some of my hair so I would understand the dreadful, desolate feeling others have when faced with this loss.

One Saturday morning I hopped into my car and drove the three minutes it takes to get to the beauty shop. Hazel, the owner, greeted me with one of her usual comments about my hair's disheveled condition! "Did you come in an ambulance?" or "Were you hit by a truck?" or perhaps, "Too bad we don't have a backdoor!" I can dish it right back: "People ask me every day where I get my hair done." I pause to make her think it's a compliment. "They want to make sure they don't come here by accident."

Unlike the newfangled shops where boys and girls prance around in tight stretch pants, swing shirts, and hair moussed up to heaven, Brookmeade Beauty Shop is just an ordinary place for neighborhood women to get the same old hairdo week after week and pay less than ten dollars. There's not even an *e* on the end of shop, much less a shampoo girl, and there are no fancy name pronunciations for Hazel, Pat, Brenda, or Ann.

My daughter goes to one of those places that has an awning out to there with a la-di-da name on it: Le Bon Ton? Rumours? or Monsieur Riqué—whose real name is probably Ricky.

"Thees ees not hair . . . I make eet hair!" says Gar-doun (perhaps Gordon?) "Ze freenge (fringe? bangs?) needs a treem (trim?)" One day Dana's curiosity got the better of her. "Gardoun, where were you born? Where do you come from?" she inquired.

"Tullahoma," he answered in the same manner he might have said "Par-ee!" Tullahoma is a small town a hundred miles from Nashville.

The truth of the matter is, even if I were bald as a billiard ball, I'd still go to Brookmeade just to visit my friends there. After twenty years of sharing the ups and downs of life, these women truly are my friends.

You find out stuff in a beauty shop. Like the best diet— no one there has lost weight on it and no one ever will, but it's the best! Recipes are handed out as freely as advice for a failing marriage or a problem daughter-in-law. If I were a politician I'd sit around a beauty shop for a few days and save money on a political analyst.

It's free therapy! Both physical and mental. In some ways a good hairdresser is more important than a good doctor . . . or lawyer . . . or psychologist! While most customers are soft-faced, grandmotherly types who giggle and tease, some have suffered almost as much as Liz Taylor. I've seen neurotics, alcoholics, and women so wracked with disease that they must be wheelchaired in and lifted to the shampoo bowl. When they leave, they have a new lease on life, not just because of a fresh hairdo, but because someone catered to their needs, listened to their complaints, and massaged their scalps. It occurs to me that for some, this is the only time they are touched.

I don't want to paint Brookmeade Beauty Shop as a mini-utopia because it's not. This next bit of information is touchy. Certain dryers belong to certain ladies. Mrs. Bridwell's is the one in the corner on the left. It's not written down anywhere, it's just something we know. If you don't want one of those gentle women to turn on you, don't take her dryer! There are frequent discussions as to which *is* and which *is not* the best dryer and sometimes the discussions are as heated as the dryers themselves.

It's not always verbal in a beauty shop. You have to understand the body language too. On some days you note a rigid determination and an irrefutable look in the eye of certain patrons that says, "Don't slow me down." If eighty-year-old Heloise Mader, former principal of Gower School, is dressed to the hilt, it's because she has a plane to catch. Probably a Civitan trip.

When Mrs. Bridwell shows up in a silk blouse and her good pumps and Jessie shows up in a skirt and stockings rather than sweats and tennis shoes, it's a good indication it's bridge day and they intend to be there when the cards are dealt. When Ann Poteet has her Bible and books spread out, she's on her way to teach her Bible class. *Don't make these ladies late!*

That eventful Saturday morning, Hazel and I exchanged our sarcastic greetings, and I waited for my turn, pulling the pins from my up-do as we chatted. I noticed an unusual amount of hair attached to the pins as I laid them on the counter.

Don't think about it, I said to myself. Pat, my hairdresser, finished with her customer, motioned me to the chair, and as usual, began brushing the hairspray from my hair. I could see that something was wrong from her reflection in the mirror, and it only took a moment to figure out what it was. My hair was coming out in handfuls!

"Let's go ahead and wash it; try not to handle it too much," she suggested. With one hand she whirled my chair around so fast she practically gave me whiplash, and with the other she raised the lid on the shampoo bowl, banging it hard against the mirror. Her quick, jerky movements made me know she was upset. Her tears made me understand how much she cared.

I shut my eyes and avoided looking into the honesty of her face while she shampooed, rinsed, and as usual, wrapped my head in a towel. Surprisingly, my hair was still there. It wasn't until she began to comb through it that we realized that most of my hair had detached itself from my scalp and was matted—as though with chewing gum—to what was left.

It took two hours to comb through my hair. That day no one argued over dryers, bridge games were forgotten, and hairdressers and customers alike took turns combing and dropping the dregs into a brown paper bag. Everyone was crying but Hazel. Her way of handling life's crises is with sarcasm and humor, but neither was appropriate, so she left—simply got in her car and drove away. Later, she commented, "How can I razz you when your hair is falling out?"

After that day in the beauty shop, no more came out. It was bad enough knowing I was green, peaked, and bloated, and often so sick I could barely hold my head up.

One night I awakened with a start and sat straight up in bed. A feeling of terror gripped me. It was as though I was being stalked. My body, and even my hair, was drenched in sweat. *What is wrong? Why am I frightened?* My mind played out all the possibilities. *Will I go through the discomforts of chemotherapy only to find out it hasn't done its job? Will I die? Might I be bedridden and a burden to my family? Will I see Dana graduate from college—Mindy, from high school? Will I be around for their weddings? Will I know my grandchildren?*

The night terrors began to happen regularly, sometimes more than once a night. Often I would fall asleep at my normal time and awaken less than an hour later to spend the rest of the night in panic. Then another problem arose. Each time I would awaken, my head would feel as though it were full of swarming bees. This only created more anxiety. *I'm going to die soon! The cancer has gone to my brain . . . Dear God, I'd rather die right now than face this fear!*

When I mentioned my problems to my doctor, he pronounced them normal. "It's normal to have problems sleeping," he explained, "and the swarming in your head is called *formication* and is a result of the strong medication." This he said while writing a prescription for more medicine! A *mild relaxer,* he called it. For a few nights it worked and I slept like a baby, but soon the problem returned. With the doctor's permission, I increased the dosage and again it helped. The next time, I increased the dosage on my own.

By summer, I was beside myself. *I have to find an answer, I'm going crazy,* I thought. *Perhaps I can get myself together while I'm in California.* (Our company coordinates much of the production for the Christian Booksellers Convention, which was in Anaheim that year.) *Hopefully working those fifteen-hour days will make me so tired I'll sleep when night comes.*

One day during the convention, my friend Donna Fisher asked if I could find time to meet with June Wark, a mutual acquaintance. June had been my Avon lady years before when we lived in the same Chicago suburb. I'd bought practically all her products, hoping they would make me as beautiful as she was. I'd lost track of her (she now lived in California) and I was delighted to hear from her again.

We met in a lounge near the exhibit floor and unlike the old June, who could lay the lipstick on the line, she was beating around the bush left and right. "I don't know if I should bother you with this . . . I'm slightly embarrassed . . . Obviously I wanted to see you . . . but besides that . . . I think I'm supposed to tell you something." She certainly had my curiosity piqued, to say the least. *Spit it out June!* I thought to myself.

"I think God is nudging me to say this . . . but . . . well, let me tell you my story. Ten years ago I had cancer and God healed me . . . but that's not the issue. It was the fear I couldn't deal with! I would wake up in the night in complete terror. I didn't want to *live* it was so bad. A friend of mine came to me and said, *June, I'm going to pray for you. I'm going to ask God to lift your fear. I won't stop praying till He answers.* Sue, I can tell you the minute and the hour my fear lifted! In fact, I was running the vacuum cleaner. I just felt free and I knew it was gone!" She paused and leaned forward and touched me, "Sue, am I supposed to be that person in your life? The person who prays till the fear stops?" She paused and smiled her winning Avon smile. "I think I am!"

When I arrived back in Nashville there was a gift waiting for me, from my friend Kate Rupert. When I unwrapped it I discovered a beautifully framed poem that still hangs on my bedroom wall.

FOOTPRINTS

There was a man who died, and he reviewed the footsteps he had taken in his life.

He looked down and noticed that all over the mountains and difficult places that he had traveled there was one set of footprints; but over the plains and down the hills, there were two sets of footprints, as if someone had walked by his side.

He turned to Christ and said,

"There is something I don't understand. Why is it that down the hills and over the smooth and easy places You have walked by my side; but, here over the rough and difficult places I have walked alone, for I see in those areas there is just one set of footprints."

Christ turned to the man and said,

"It is that while your life was easy I walked along your side; but here, where the walking was hard and the paths were difficult, was the time you needed ME most, and that is why I carried you." Author unknown

The words were a confirmation of June's message, that I couldn't manage alone, that I needed God's divine help to take the next step and let go of the pills. When I did, I slept like a baby, and the terrors never returned.

My yellow cat stuck with me through it all. For a while after my treatment was over, he would meet us at the door, lead us to the bedroom, leap on the bed, and look at us expectantly. He seemed to be saying, "Come on, let's be sick some more!"

One day Ya didn't come when we called. We searched the woods. He never went far. Every day after that we hoped as we came up the drive. Finally I knew he was gone forever, and I wrote "Eulogy to Ya." A eulogy to a cat, you say? Yes, a eulogy to a cat!

Dear Ya,

　　I guess you're really gone. This morning a fluff of your yellow-orange fur skitted across the driveway, but when I reached for it, a gust of wind swept it up to the sky. That's when I knew you wouldn't be coming back. I miss you and hope your last moments were peaceful. I would have liked to comfort you as you comforted me so many times.

I remember the day we got you. You were just a ball of yellow fluff in Uncle Jon's hand. Dana and Mindy named you Yata which is the Greek word for cat, because Grandma had been to Greece and learned that word. She told us how she laughed when she heard the Greek ladies call, "Yata, yata," and saw their cats come running. We thought it was funny too.

You grew big and beautiful, and although you "frowned" a lot, we knew you loved your family and enjoyed the woods on "your" property. We even caught you smelling the flowers on occasion.

There's probably not a cat heaven, but if there is, I suppose you've met up with Goodie (Baddie is probably in that other place), Smokey, the Pirate, Don Derk of Don Day, and my beloved Agamemnon. Perhaps you're all comparing notes on little girls you've known.

Chapter 6

Statistics?
I'm the
Only Me!

A ll women should be Mexican and illiterate." A doctor said that to me not long after my mastectomy. We were discussing whether or not a woman should know the statistics of her prognosis. I was appalled! My daughters accuse me of being confrontive in such a situation: "When Mother takes issue with someone, she gets right in their face and sticks her finger up their nose!" An exaggeration, of course! However, had this not been a phone conversation, I might have been tempted to do just that. I merely shouted, "You can't mean that!"

His remark seemed sexist and very much like a racial slur, but I did my best to take his frame of reference into account. He lived and worked in New Mexico, and he treated many Mexican women who were illiterate and unable to pay. I knew he was compassionate, caring, and tops in oncology. I listened.

"People don't need to know their chances. Most patients hear the negative when it comes to ratios. I may be wrong, but I think I see people die because they hear the wrong number. I just wish they were too ignorant to ask." I could hear the anguish in his voice.

His way of counteracting the negative statistics was ignorance. My friend Trish, who owns a cosmetic company called

Aloette, believes we counteract the negative with a life attitude. I tend to agree. Sales in Trish's company are accomplished through home party demonstrations, and once a year
the women get together for a sales meeting. They see new
products, learn sales tips, and share success stories. The con-
ference was in Nashville not long ago, and Trish invited me to
come to the hotel for the final meeting.

Wow! Such energy! Such enthusiasm! Three hundred
women excited about beauty products. They cheered, they
clapped, they jumped—some even stood on their chairs and
jumped—and they cried. If their children acted like that, these
women undoubtedly would be screaming, "Settle down this
minute or you can go to your room!"

The program was packed with opportunities for the
women to exhibit their ardent zeal. As the meeting progressed, with awards and recognitions, the crowd energy ac-
celerated to what I thought was its peak. I hadn't seen
anything, though, until they introduced Trish.

"And now, ladies, what you've all been waiting for, our
founder, our leader, our motivator, Trr-iiiish!" She entered
the rear of the auditorium and made her way down the center
aisle, waving to the crowd, stopping now and then to touch
the hands that reached for her—the spotlight catching the sequins on her dress, like the Christmas tree in Rockefeller Center. I sat there spellbound as Trish spoke.

"Have you looked into the sky and seen birds flying in
formation?" Trish asked. The ladies nodded.

"Have you noticed they fly in that *V* formation?" She
swept across the stage making a *V* in the air with her finger.
They nodded again.

"Have you noticed that one side of the *V* is longer?"
This time they moved forward on their chairs, and their whole
bodies nodded. Her voice softened to a whisper.

"Do you want to know why one side is longer?" Oh,
they did, they did; they've lived for this moment.

"Because one side has more birds!" There was a rush of
laughter, but it was cut short as she continued to speak. They
didn't want to miss a word.

"I'm a very basic person and what I have to tell you is very basic. *I'm going to tell you how you can be rich!*" A cacophony of cheers! Her showmanship down pat, Trish paused, then in a you'll-never-believe-this tone of voice, she began her story, "Less than fifteen years ago, I"—she laid her diamond laden hand on her glittering bosom—"was giving the cosmetic parties. My husband and I had just bought a new home without selling the old one, and the expenses of two homes were mounting by the moment. My parents loaned us $10,000, but that only increased the burden." Trish walked the stage with her head bowed. Her audience was with her.

"Then the unexpected." Pause. "I had to have emergency surgery!" The audience felt the knife. You could see it in each face.

"And on top of all of that . . ." the audience was holding its breath, waiting to know what could be worse. ". . . as I left the hospital, the doctor told me I couldn't drive a car for a month." They sighed in unison.

"Well, ladies, how could I have makeup parties when I couldn't drive? And how could we make it through this financial crisis when I couldn't have those parties?" I could almost hear those women ponder. Trish bowed her head again and then lifted it, smiling. "Ladies, the doctor said I couldn't *drive,* he didn't say I couldn't *give parties!* I simply found someone else to do the driving . . ." I turned to look at the nonplussed faces that said, "Why didn't I think of that?"

". . . and do you know, I had the biggest month in sales I ever had!" She quoted a figure. "The very biggest!" In one great swell the audience rose to its feet. Cheering! Clapping! Once again Trish moved in close to the microphone for the zinger.

"Ladies, what do *you* hear?"

With that introduction, Trish set the stage to address the plague of her company and every other company—negative thinking. *And* it's what every cancer patient—or heart patient or accident victim or substance abuse overcomer—must surmount. "Women should be Mexican and illiterate" was the doctor's way of counteracting negative thinking. "What they don't know won't hurt them." I prefer Trish's way. It's an attitude adjustment.

Another story, courtesy of Trish, brings the subject down to the nitty-gritty. It seems a seventy-year-old woman in New York, named Josie Green, was dying of cancer. One day she managed to get out of bed and walk to the corner. She passed a neighbor who said, "Josie, you look good today," so she thought, *Well, maybe since I don't look so bad, I'll fix myself up a bit and go to the theater tonight.* So she went to the theater.

Afterward someone walked up to her and said, "Josie, you look ten years younger." The next day Josie said to herself, *If I look ten years younger, I'll just dye my hair and get around more.*

The next time she went out someone said to her, "Josie, you don't look a day over forty." *Well if I look that good,* she thought, *I'll move to California!* She moved to California, met a twenty-five-year-old man, and married him.

The next day she was hit by a car and died. Was Josie ever mad! The angels had to drag her across the floor of heaven to the throne of God, where she proceeded to give God "what for!"

When God could finally get a word in edgewise, He said, "Josie, I'm sorry! I made a mistake. I didn't mean for you to die! You looked so good I didn't recognize you!"

God doesn't make mistakes, of course; neither does He lose track of His charges. But I can just picture old Josie out there in California in her tight leather miniskirt and hot pink halter. She heard the right things, all right.

I wish everyone I talk to could hear the good stuff instead of bad statistics. One woman asked her doctor what her chances for survival were. When he told her they were 70 percent for a ten-year survival—based on the number of malignant lymph nodes—she was confident she would survive.

Yet the next day she told me she was going to die. "I have a gut feeling I'm not going to live," she said. When I asked her why she had gone from hope*ful* to hope*less* in a twenty-four-hour period, she told me she'd read different statistics from her doctor's, called him, and insisted he tell her the truth. He admitted her case fell on the line between two sets of numbers, and he had chosen to give her the more hopeful answer. It seemed she was more comfortable with the negative outlook than the positive.

My friend, Paul Keckley, is a marketing research guru—a numbers man. If it can't be proved on paper or on the computer screen, it can't happen. I read about a man named Irving who, like Paul, was a statistician. He developed cancer, and his oncologist told him his chances which were not good. From then on he refused to fight for his life.

He said, "I've spent my life making predictions based on statistics. Statistics show I'm supposed to die. If I don't die, my whole life doesn't make sense." The story goes that he went home and died.

Paul is different; he has invested his life in making predictions based on statistics and he's rigid in that pursuit; but he also believes in a personal God who does personal miracles. So do I. I *am* one.

Not long after I began treatment, I saw an article in the paper that said studies had been done proving that state of mind has nothing to do with the prognosis and survival rate of a cancer patient. I didn't believe it then, and I don't believe it now.

Once I heard my chances, I decided to disregard them. In many ways, I fell perfectly into the tabulations. "Let's see; she's forty-five, white, female, 5'8" tall, weight—*bleep*. Hmmm, let's throw in some medical stuff . . . metastatic adenocarcinoma present in fourteen of twenty-six ancillary lymph nodes. Well, looks like this one won't be around too long!"

I'm convinced the computer can't capture my exacts. I am the only, *the very only,* Suzanne Davis Buchanan, and I come from a long line of sturdy progenitors. Those Ensmingers, McKnights, Nelsons, and Braleys lived long, healthy lives, and there are a million, maybe a trillion, other minuscule things that the calculations can never take into account: what I eat and drink; how much I sleep and exercise; or how often I laugh or make love. Neither can it know that I am wrapped in the loving care of Wayne, Dana, and Melinda, and am prayed for daily by Jimmy, Lynn, Evelyn, Bob, Joy, John, Betsy, Paul, Rhonda, Marsha, Chuck, Tommy, and Phyllis— my Sunday night group—all of whom believe in miracles! And furthermore, I doubt there will ever be a computer program that can look into the future to see whether a person takes the prescribed medication or flushes it.

Chapter 7

Some Words
Should Be
Whispered

My name is Edna Puckett. You don't know me. I'm just one of the little people." She pouts. Then she leans toward someone in the front row and in her most abrasive old lady voice asks, "You can't see my underwear, can you?" The word *underwear* is spoken in a loud whisper, and her eyes dart as though someone might come out of the woodwork to arrest her for saying it. Aunt Edna has opinions about anything and everything.

"Don't get me started," she challenges. But it's too late; she's off and running, waxing eloquent about whatever comes to her mind. Those know-it-alls with tongue depressors in their pockets and stethoscopes dangling around their necks or those *deee*-mon rock-and-rollers who travel in buses with darkened windows. She'll even take on the telephone company. She's had it with those television ads: "I've had about all of this *reach out and touch* stuff I can stomach!"

Every family has a "character" person (mine was Aunt Annie, Wayne's Aunt Naomi). These individuals are the perpetuators of the family name and the preservers and translators of family history. Though they usually lack training, they are at once psychologist, physician, parent, pastor, and philosopher, freely dispensing unsolicited advice in large doses, accompanied by the vigorous shaking of an index finger.

Aunt Edna isn't a real character anymore than Mrs. Van-dertweezers. My friend Joy created her for a church skit and insisted I was the one to play the part.

Aunt Edna didn't go away after the play. Every so often someone calls to ask if she's available for a birthday party, and I pull her out of the bag—knotty little gray wig, sensible old-lady shoes, knee-high stockings, navy polyester skirt, red blouse, and ratty white sweater with a pin that says, "Over the hill, not under it!" Her rouge is uneven, and her lipstick is smeared almost to her nose.

Her spiritual "gift," she says, is the gift of criticism, and she's quick to tell the minister, whom she calls "preacher," she likes the *beginning* of his sermon and she likes the *end* of his sermon. Then, with a laugh, she suggests, "How 'bout getting the two closer together!" She wants to know all the church gossip, so she can "pray more intelligently."

Edna gets a little more wound up at a party than she does in the church's fellowship hall. She confides, "When I was young, I was a hot little number . . . I once set a young man's tie on fire!" or "In my day, I was kissed more times than the pope's ring."

Aunt Edna believes words such as *cancer, underwear, breasts,* and *sex* should be spoken in a whisper. Her generation wouldn't think of saying such words aloud!

My generation wasn't quite so conservative. As teenagers we spoke the word *sex* aloud and were curious about it, but most of us wouldn't have risked sex outside of marriage, mainly for fear of pregnancy. We also had our parents' wrath to contend with. In those days, it wasn't a case of your parents' grounding you—they would *kill* you!

We didn't have the privilege of attending a class to discuss sex or finding a counselor to help us through it; we simply didn't do it. In fact, it wasn't something we even thought about much because the opportunities weren't there. For one thing, our parents stayed up until our dates left. My mother sometimes even walked my boyfriend to the door! "Bye, Ray! Don't let the cat in when you leave. Drive carefully, and thank your mom for the yellow tomatoes."

About the only hugging and kissing we did was in cars. In the fifties, cars were our drugs! All we thought and talked about. Who had one? What color was it? How fast would it go, and how many people could it hold? Some guys (rarely girls) were lucky enough to borrow the family car occasionally, and a few actually owned one. In those days, a teenager's car was always packed like a jar of olives.

I still love to get into a car that's been closed up overnight and take that first deep breath. If it were possible to have bottled the car smells of my youth, you could blindfold me and I'd pass the sniffing test—tell you which bottle held the smell of the interior of Ray's pink and black Ford, identify that of Gary's yellow convertible, and, without a doubt, know the distinctive smell of Harold's Jeep. I have good memories of cars packed full of laughing teenagers. I also have memories of long, lingering kisses in the backseat of someone's car, interrupted by teeth crashing together because of those bumpy West Virginia roads.

When I became a college freshman, my high school naivete, faded rapidly. One of my first college dates was a tall, dark, handsome trumpet major who gave me the impression that I should feel fortunate to be his choice for the evening. He didn't even kiss me; he went straight for the breasts!

My exit line was, "Okay Columbus, you've discovered enough!" I made the mistake of telling my daughters about this experience once when we were discussing sex and they never forgot it. We still say those words and laugh.

That experience awakened an uneasy feeling in me. Having someone touch my breasts was worse than having seventh-grade boys look at them.

As a married woman, I learned that breasts were for admiring and caressing, a satisfying part of the lovemaking process. Just when I'd begun to accept and enjoy my breasts, one was cut off.

How could I not worry that my husband would reject me, think of me as not being whole or sexy? In the hospital I could pull the robes and bedjackets tightly around me, but coming home was a different story.

The first night I went into the dark closet to put on my gown. I pulled out a beautiful floor-length one with a lacy built-in bra and quickly stuffed the left side with socks. I looked in the mirror as I stepped from the closet. *Not bad,* I thought, *Not bad at all.* With a flair I got into my side of the bed. Wayne smiled.

With no hesitation at all he took me in his arms and made love to me, cautiously but passionately. That night an unspoken agreement went into effect between the two of us; for the next year, the nightgown stayed on during lovemaking. I chose to be private about my body, and he respected my decision. Not long before my reconstructive surgery I showed him my scar. He reached out and touched it and looked into my eyes.

"I'll bet you'll be glad to get that fixed," he said and turned back to his book. I can honestly say, my mastectomy didn't threaten the intimacy of our marriage. If anything, it made us closer.

Every case is not like mine. I know of several men who physically walked away from their wives after a mastectomy. I know some who walked away emotionally. Women ask, "How can this surgery *not* affect our lovemaking? How can I go along as though nothing is wrong?" Men ask, "How can I show her it's okay, that I don't want it to affect our sex life?" Men sometimes ask more questions than women: "Shall I pretend it never happened? Should we laugh? Should we cry?"

A very good place to get answers to questions like these is the American Cancer Society's A New Beginning program, which meets regularly to give the breast cancer patient information and emotional support.

Husbands, daughters, and friends are invited and often come. There is usually a program or speaker, but the real purpose of the group is to meet the woman where she is, at whatever stage of emotion, and be there for her.

Because of my busy schedule, I've attended only a couple of times. Both times I intended to duck in and out, simply to hear the speaker, but both times I was pulled into the camaraderie and spirit of the group.

The first time I attended, the meeting was led by a woman named Josie, young, with beautiful, black, almost iridescent skin. I thought to myself, *This woman's never had a bad day in her life. She's being paid to do this; she's a staff member.*

Josie opened the meeting by suggesting we get acquainted. "We'll go around the room, tell our names and where we are right now in our cancer journey. First of all, I'm Josie, and it's been almost seven years since I had a modified radical mastectomy. I had fourteen bad lymph nodes. I was twenty-four when it happened and didn't know a thing about cancer till it hit home. I thought I was going to die. Then I said, 'No, I've always thought positively. You're half way there if you can think positively—I can lick it. I have the best doctors in the world, and my belief in God is strong.' I just kept saying, 'You can lick it!' It wasn't easy.

"At the same time I was taking chemotherapy, I was taking radiation—upstairs for chemo, downstairs for radiation— day after day! I had a year of chemo and thirty radiation treatments. Five years later I had reconstruction and now I'm well and healthy." She glowed!

Each woman in the first row stood and told her name and the status of her battle with cancer. Some had been cancer-free for years, some were in treatment and hanging on to the hope that they, like Josie, would lick it! In the second row a woman stood, spoke her name, and burst into tears. We waited for her to regain her composure.

"I thought I was well. I did everything they told me to do, but I've just had a recurrence. It's back. My cancer's back!" We waited in uncomfortable silence, punctuated only by an occasional loud, gut-wrenching sob. Without a moment's hesitation, Josie walked across the room and stood by her side. With her beautiful hands she stroked the woman's face, wiping her tears. The meeting came to a dead halt. The most important thing at that moment was not to hear a speaker, see a film, or listen to a tape, but to comfort. As long as the tears fell—and it seemed an eternity—Josie's glistening hands wiped them away. I'll never forget that moment. It is a strong mental image that appears every time I'm asked, "Just what *does* The American Cancer Society do?"

The question of intimacy after breast cancer often comes up at these meetings, and the volunteers are equipped to help. I asked Donna, another American Cancer Society volunteer, "You've talked to a lot of women, and men too. What gets couples through this mastectomy ordeal with their sexual relationships intact?"

"I think if you start out with a close, intimate relationship you have a better chance, but on the other hand, I've heard of it working the other way; couples having a tenuous relationship can be brought together by the trauma of a mastectomy. I guess there's no pat answer."

As for me and my husband, we found that humor greatly helped ease the intimacy problem. Often what we couldn't talk about, we could laugh about. After my first program of chemotherapy—which began in the hospital—Wayne surprised me with a trip to Puerto Rico, one of the most wonderful, intimate times we ever spent together.

We stayed in an elegant hotel and every day got up late, ate a leisurely breakfast, sunned by the ocean, walked, talked, took naps, dressed for dinner, and strolled the hotel, "people watching," one of our favorite things to do.

My husband made two comments that week that many people would think strange, but for me, they were a turning point in our postoperative relationship, which assured me that things hadn't changed between us at all. One night he bought tickets to what was described as a "Las Vegas Show" in the hotel where we were staying.

Although we weren't warned ahead of time, the dance extravaganza finale featured bare-breasted women. At first, Wayne was all eyes. Then suddenly, aware of the strangeness of the circumstances, he leaned close, took my hand and without missing a beat, said; "I was just counting . . . they all have two! Let's go."

On another day, I teasingly asked him, "Do you think

you can love me now for my *mind* instead of my body?" Without flinching, he answered, "Honey, if I'd seen as much of your mind as I have your body, I'd be able to tell you!"

To some, those responses may seem unkind or even cruel. To me, they ensured our sense of humor was intact.

Recently, I was reacquainted with a distant relative at a funeral. Other than playing together once or twice—she lived in Columbus, Ohio, and I lived in Charleston—the thing I remembered most vividly about Janice was that I, as a child, wore her hand-me-down clothes: Every year or so a box came and there would be five or six beautiful, almost new dresses.

After the funeral we went back to my uncle's home for dinner. In the course of the afternoon, Janice shared with me the fact she too had had breast cancer. With a twinkle in her eye she told me she wore a homemade prosthesis—her experience with store-bought ones was unsatisfactory. She explained how she had come up with the ingenious idea of filling a piece of nylon stocking with birdseed, and stuffing it in the pocket she had sewn in her bra.

"Works great," she said. Then with a slight blush, she added, "Tom says you can look in the sky and tell when I'm comin' by the great trail of birds following me!" I knew by the humor that Tom, like Wayne, had helped his wife feel comfortable about a very touchy subject.

Many women have shared with me their first sexual experience after a mastectomy. Some tell of renewed romantic interest; others tell stories best described as nightmares. I went to visit Marlene, at the request of a mutual friend. Marlene, who was unmarried, was belligerent about the subject of reconstructive surgery.

"Why should I have my breasts rebuilt just to make some man happy?" she said. "When I meet someone, he'll just have to get used to it!"

One day she called to tell me she'd gone away on a singles weekend, and after getting chummy with one of the male attendees—and drunk in the process—she ended up in his bed. The man, reaching for a breast and finding instead a thick scar, literally jumped from the bed in horror, practically throwing her to the floor in the process. Marlene didn't learn her lesson; she repeated the experience several times over. The last time I spoke with her she said, "I've had some real bad experiences with sex." It didn't occur to her that a one-night stand isn't the place to find a sympathetic mate.

Kitty came to visit me right after my mastectomy and was appalled that I would consider "putting myself under the knife" again to have reconstructive surgery. "I had a double mastectomy years ago and my husband loves me just like I am. We've had no problems at all, no problems at all." She brought the subject up several times during her visit. Years later I hired a decorator who had worked with Kitty. I explained I'd had a bad year—having had a mastectomy, chemo, and reconstructive surgery—and wanted to spruce up the living room a bit.

"Be glad you had reconstructive surgery," he said. "I work with this woman named Kitty who decided against it. She and her husband had trouble from day one, and it hasn't ended yet!"

Both Marlene and Kitty were unrealistic and had adopted an almost combative attitude toward their circumstances. I'm glad that's not the norm. Donna, my friend from the American Cancer Society, tells me the "unofficial" survey at A New Beginning says most relationships tend to improve during this life-shattering experience, and my own unofficial survey seems to agree.

A young teacher told me she'd had small breasts to begin with so it hardly made a difference. Later her husband repeated the same story. Both told of a new, deeper intimacy than they'd had before, and their eyes told me this was true.

Last week a thirty-seven-year-old woman called from California. We'd never met, but I've discovered sometimes it's much easier to talk to a stranger, miles away, than it is to talk to a friend or family member. After a mastectomy Beverly is in the process of finishing up her chemotherapy. She has two small children and her husband is out of work. She confided that her relationship with her husband, which was tenuous before the mastectomy, was now quite strong. She has no plans for reconstructive surgery.

Joanie did as I did—chose not to let her mate see her naked body after her mastectomy. She told me she kept her body covered, wore teddies or gowns, and locked the bathroom door when she bathed. One day she forgot to lock the door and Will walked in. Quickly she tried to cover herself with the washcloth as she begged him to get out! Undeterred, he moved to the edge of the tub, knelt, took her in his arms, and said, "I love *you,* not your breasts. When will you understand?"

"He cried and I cried and it all ran together . . . *my* tears, *his* tears, and the bath water!" she told me. What a wonderful way to wash away the fear and uncertainty!

Chapter 8

When It Rains, It Pours

W hen it rains, it pours." Noah's wife said that! It was the thirty-ninth day she'd been on that creaky ark, with all those sneezing, sniveling relatives. Everyone was out of clothes; the ones she'd washed five days before were still wet. She was down to the last of the food supplies, and she'd had all she could stand of restless, smelly, wet animals. She didn't dare turn her back for fear of being kicked by a kangaroo, swatted by a lion, or stepped on by a rhinoceros. She'd been a healthy woman when she stepped on that boat, now she was as claustrophobic and paranoid as she could get, with a permanent case of vertigo to boot!

Noah's wife never realized it, but her words caught on like loincloths after the fall of man. All through early biblical history people repeated it. Sarah said to Abraham, "Abraham, it seems to me, when it rains, it pours. Does it seem that way to you?" And Lot said to Lot's wife, "Wife, did you ever notice; when it rains, it pours?"

Read Genesis if you want to read about major life trauma. These people were not living balanced, healthy lives! They were not in good relationships. Most of them were living out of suitcases, traveling on donkeys, and sleeping in tents, which is bound to predispose a family to dysfunction. Each time they stopped, they built an altar. Compulsion, if I ever saw it. Maybe an applauded addiction!

It was a driven society full of risk-takers, going to war at the drop of a hat and having to survive all those physiological illnesses without a PPO, HMO, or Convenient Care Center. Just learning about circumcision for the first time must have been a jolt to the psychological persona!

Friends and family members were dying left and right and yet they were without the benefit of grief and anger books. And famines were apparently endured without the help of rock concerts, foreign aid, or Willie Nelson!

Check out that first book in the Bible, if you think things are messed up today—a wife pretending to be her husband's sister, daughters having babies by their father, people being tricked into marriages, a woman turning to salt, angels fighting off homosexuals, unexplainable dreams, a brother killing his brother, brothers selling a brother, and more—strong indications of a need for reparenting due to negative messages as a result of generational, relational fallout!

Down through history when the load became almost too heavy to bear, when everything bad seemed to happen at once, people said it. Mrs. Noah's catchy slogan was even picked up by the salt company. And folks still say it today: "When it rains, it pours!"

I visit a woman with breast cancer and she tells me her insurance lapsed a month before her illness or that her son had a car accident or her unmarried daughter is pregnant or her husband just lost his job—sometimes all of the above!

"If it were *just* cancer, I could handle it," she tells me, "but it's all these other things happening at the same time!" When it comes to problems, it truly does seem they arrive in torrents. It was true for me. The year of my mastectomy and chemotherapy, my downpour centered on my mother's illness.

"Anything that makes you that sick couldn't be good for you," Mother's husband Jim had said about her chemotherapy treatments. Soon she was parroting his words, and not long after that she stopped going altogether. It was hard for our family to believe our life-loving mother would give up so easily. It seemed so unlike her.

I knew she wondered where I was, why I hadn't come during her most recent setback. I called her each day, with the exception of the day of my surgery, and tried to cheer her up. I could barely hear her voice as she lapsed in and out of consciousness.

As soon as the doctor would let me, I made arrangements to fly to West Palm Beach where Mother's husband, Jim, would pick me up and take me to Boca Raton Hospital. I hoped to spend the time with my mother, even planned to stay the night in her room.

I felt that given the chance, Jim would manipulate me. I knew the pattern from past experience: He would take me to the hospital and stand impatiently on one foot, then the other, while I visited with Mother; then after an hour or so he'd suggest we leave so she could rest. If I wanted to see Mother again in the evening, he would give me a short no-questions-asked answer: "It's not necessary!"

Before my trip, Wayne called ahead to pave the way. "Please take Sue to the hospital and leave her there. She wants to spend the time with her mother. Don't insist she go out to eat. Let her pick up something at the hospital, and please don't involve her in any decisions; she's not up to it." Jim was planning to move Mother to a nursing home and had suggested we spend our time shopping for the right facility. My brothers were both on call for decision making.

As I flew south, the lump in my stomach was not from my medication or worry for Mother, but from the dread of dealing with Jim. Walking out through the jetway, I could see his smiling face, eagerly waiting. A pang of guilt ran through me as I thought of the pain this poor man had suffered. His first wife had died a long, slow death from cancer, and now he was losing Mother, whom he called the love of his life.

Before we were even on the expressway, Jim began, "We have a lot of work to do, many decisions to be made. I hope you're in no hurry to get to the hospital. I have several appointments lined up." I gulped.

"We need to plan the funeral while you're here," he continued as he pulled the car off the road and into a parking lot. I wondered why we were stopping in front of a large white house. *Probably a restaurant,* I thought. The big funeral home sign didn't register. My brain was numb.

"Dear." He always called me that. "I've picked a casket. It's quite lovely. It has a peach lining. Your mother would like it. She's always liked peach. I want you to see it . . . approve it."

Like a zombie I got out of the car. His hand under my elbow, he swept me up the steps. The door opened, automatically it seemed, and there stood Lurch of "The Addams Family" TV fame, except his suit was white instead of black. His smile was the same.

Lurch led us to a large room full of caskets. All colors, all sizes, all prices. Jim took my arm and guided me across the room, stopping in front of a pale gray number with a peach lining. Sure enough, it was the perfect choice! Just what Mother would have chosen herself and sure enough, I behaved just as Mother would have wanted me to. I didn't scream profane words or scratch out Jim's eyes or kick Lurch in the groin. Instead, I smiled sweetly, ran my hands over the satin (probably acetate) lining, admired the styling, nodded my head in agreement and said that yes, it was probably the loveliest casket I'd ever seen and perfect for my mother. Just perfect!

Perhaps it is the right thing to do, plan for Mother's death, I thought as we drove away. *After all, it's only natural Jim would want me to have a say in the decisions.* Little did I imagine, it would be nine long months before we would actually need the peach-lined casket.

But right then, nothing would do but that we stop for lunch. After lunch—a lunch I didn't want—he took me to the hospital, and I tried to ignore him as I visited with Mother. As I had anticipated, he stood on one foot, then the other. She was barely conscious, but I knew she felt my touch, and her questioning eyes met mine as I talked to her. Jim was in a hurry. He had things he wanted to do, and I was part of his plan.

We visited the three nursing homes. At the third, I discovered he'd already given them a check for the first month! I hoped against hope the actual move would take place after I was back in Nashville, but that was not to be. I soon found that Jim's plans were to move Mother the very next day so I could help him.

"It's not necessary," was Jim's response when I asked to be taken to see Mother that evening on our way home from dinner. "What you need is a good night's sleep, dear." I knew him well enough to know that his answer was final and making a scene would give him the opportunity to condescend to me: "Oh, you poor thing! You *are* upset! You really do need a good night's sleep!"

I'd bitten my lip almost bloody to keep from speaking my mind throughout the day. I'd kept my mouth shut when he vetoed a visit to the hospital, but the next thing that happened made me lose it completely!

We no sooner were in the door of the condominium, than he turned to me and said, "Your mother won't be needing her clothes anymore. I want you to go through her closet and get things ready for me to take to the resale shop tomorrow." I quietly followed him to Mother's closet, and when I saw the rows of familiar dresses, I came unglued. I reached for the first dress, pulled it out, hanger and all, and flung it on the bed shouting, "I bought this! I bought this! And this, and this!" Dress after dress flew through the air. Then I turned to him, and with my finger practically up his nose, I spat out, "You . . aren't . . getting . . rid . . of . . *my* . . mother's . . clothes!" I saw a glimmer of terror in his eyes. "I'll pack them and take them to Nashville, but you're not selling *anything!*"

The next day, we moved Mother from the hospital to the nursing home. It seemed more than I could bear, to see her poor painracked body jostled from bed to stretcher to ambulance and to bed again.

After she was settled in her new surroundings, I insisted Jim leave us alone. I picked Mother's shrunken, cadaver-like body up in my arms and held her and rocked her. Her eyes never left mine, questioning. Suddenly we were both crying, our tears mingling and our bodies shaking with great heaves and soundless sobs. I didn't dare open my mouth for fear of blurting out the truth, that I too had cancer. Perhaps she knew. Sometimes mothers just know!

My last visit to Florida before Mother's death was peaceful. Wayne insisted I rent a car so as not to depend on Jim. Why hadn't we thought of it sooner? For the most part, Jim left me alone. I sat by Mother's bedside each day and chattered, knowing that she could hear me even though she had no strength to respond. I told her in great detail about our beautiful little Cara Jane and the joy she brought to all of us. I reminisced.

"Remember Daddy's gourds? How we always had to brag on them? Do you think they're still growing up over the garage on Mathews Avenue? Know what, Mama? I still have a basketful of those gourds in my family room."

I assured her that my brothers and I were in loving, nourishing marriages. I told her how very close the six of us—Jon and Beck, Joe and Carolyn, and Wayne and I—had become, that I thought of my sisters-in-law (including Wayne's sister Pard) as the sisters I never had. I knew Mother would die soon and I wanted her to take comfort in the fact she had done a good job, that everything was fine with her children.

Recently, I've learned that letting your dying loved one go—saying "Everything is fine, I release you"—is a good thing to do. Just last night, Joy, Gloria, and I sat on the bedroom floor as Gloria told us about the moments just before her mother's death. We knew Dorothy as a spunky, outspoken, in-charge grandmother who ruled with a firm but loving hand as she took over Gloria's house and children almost every weekend when Gloria was on the road singing and speaking.

Dorothy had been hospitalized for months. The pain and indignities of her illness were unspeakable yet she couldn't seem to let go. "She was fighting to stay alive," Gloria told us.

"Finally one day it dawned on me she was probably fighting because she knew we expected it of her. She had been a fighter all her life and that's all she knew to do. I said, 'Mother, you don't have to fight anymore. You've been the best mother in the world. I'm fine. Evelyn is fine.' I picked her up in my arms and told her we could make it without her and that she didn't have to struggle anymore. After that she took four or five breaths and she was gone."

One day while I was with Mother, old friends from Charleston came to visit. The few people who had visited before barely glanced at her, spoke quietly to me, and left as quickly as possible. Not Bill and Sylvia! They ran to Mother's side, took her hands in theirs, and spoke directly to her. "Mary Jane, we're so excited for you! You're going home! You're going to heaven! You're going to see Maynard." My daddy. "Oh, tell him 'hello' for us! Mary Jane, you'll be well . . . and it will be so wonderful."

Suddenly I was no longer sad. Mother wasn't dying. She was going home. And yes! She would be well! She would see Daddy! It *would* be wonderful!

Not long before Mother's death, Dr. Solomon changed my treatment. He explained that the new protocol was more debilitating than the one I had been on and that it would most likely lower my white blood count and my resistance. I'd already experienced times when my white count was so low treatment had to be postponed. Now it would be certain to happen again. He warned about possible side effects—mouth sores, infection, and loss of hair.

"We'll give you these new drugs as long as your system can tolerate them," he said. "Then we'll go back to the original program." I remember that one drug was called Vinblastin, and after two or three treatments I thought, *Its name serves it well! It certainly is blastin' me!*

What hair I had left turned from blonde to an ugly, dull shade of steel gray. Once again my friends at the beauty shop stood by to help, but despite innumerable hours there my hair refused to respond. Pat, Hazel, Brenda, and Ann couldn't help my hair, but they always managed to lift my spirits and make me laugh at my dilemma.

All of my body odors intensified, with an added whiff of chemical. "Can't you smell that?" I'd ask my husband. "How can you bear to be near me?" He swore he didn't notice.

A couple of times I hallucinated. One night at home I felt smothered, and I wrapped myself in a quilt and walked out on the sundeck to get a breath of fresh air. It was a clear, cool, starry night, and I stretched out on the chaise longue, pulling the quilt up around my chin. I lay there for a long time looking into the sky. Up, up, up through the stars.

This must be what it feels like to be a druggie, I thought, aware of the effects of the strong medicine. *I've heard about it, but never experienced it. This must be what it feels like to trip out.*

Up, up, up through the stars. If I look closely I can see right into the laughing faces of my parents and their friends, Margarite and Capey. If I listen, I can hear them speaking.

"Capey, how are you doing on that television you're building?" my mother asks.

"There are parts everywhere—all over the house," Margarite whines. I can see the deep pockmarks on her otherwise pretty face.

"I've never seen a television *work,*" my daddy says, ". . . but if anyone can build one that works, Capey, you can." They all look down at me, in my lounge chair or on the rag rug on the floor. Wherever I am!

Then I'm floating, like a combination of swimming and flying. The stars seem to be over and under and all around me. I can look down and see myself lying in the lounge chair, but when I look, I see myself not as an adult but as a child, little more than a baby. I am lying on my back, on a rag rug, in the kitchen of my childhood home on Sixth Street in Charleston. I am holding a little pimento cheese glass full of water. Mother and Daddy and Margarite and Capey are standing above me, trying their best to convince me that drinking water while lying on my back is a bad idea.

"You can't do it, Suz," my daddy is saying. "You'll choke." I pay no attention. I tip the glass to my mouth. Water—instead of gushing over me—*sprinkles* down on me. On my face . . . in my eyes . . . on my hair.

Suddenly I am back on the chaise longue on the deck, and rain is falling on my face.

Another time—during the day—I lay on my back on the sundeck, looking into the sky. Up, up, up, perhaps to infinity. Again my sensory perception was intensified by the drugs.

I can hear the echo of a voice.

"Sue, you are wearing me out!" It's one of my great aunts—Aunt Annie or Aunt Maggie. They both sound the same. "Lie still and hush. Do you hear me?"

Up, up, up. This time into the picture that hangs above the daybed in the old home place in southern Ohio. Aunt Maggie and Aunt Annie have told me that I need to rest because I'm wearing them out. I've looked up into the picture at least a million times, but this time I'm experiencing the eerily familiar sensation of both swimming and flying. Right into the picture, I'm going. Up the gray fieldstone steps with hollyhocks and snapdragons and roses all around me. When I get to the top and walk under the archway of roses, there is a playhouse. If I go inside, there will be a winding stairway, like the one in the old home place, where my aunts rarely let me play. "Too drafty," they say.

Still I decide to play on the stairway in the playhouse. It will be the multilevel Hollywood apartment house for the fake paper dolls I cut from the Montgomery Ward catalog.

"She'll catch her death," I hear one of the aunts say, ". . in that cold, drafty stairway."

I'm looking out the window of my playhouse and I see, not the child on the daybed, but the adult me who wonders momentarily if she's caught her death from playing on the cold, drafty stairway. Otherwise why would she feel so wretched?

I pull myself out of the lounge chair and go into the house, knowing that the incident really happened—both incidents, in fact—long before I could remember, when I was a very small child. The drugs were responsible for the return of these memories.

What strikes me today is the vividness and intensity of those hallucinations and the feeling that I was understanding "truth" in life-shaking proportions. It makes me understand why a person can be bamboozled by mind-altering drugs. Under their influence, a relatively insignificant memory or thought can manifest itself in monstrous proportions.

One day I sat in my office wondering how much longer I could go on with my treatment, especially this new, more aggressive protocol. I wanted to continue as long as possible, but I could tell it was taking its toll. It was midafternoon on Friday, and I longed for the day to be over so I could "crash" for the weekend. All of a sudden my breathing became labored.

"Abby," I called to my secretary, "I'm feeling really weird, as though my breathing is being cut off."

"Let's get you to the couch," she said, guiding me in that direction.

"I know this sounds crazy, but I feel as though I'm smothering. I'm . . . dying," I said as I fell back against the pillows. I was blacking out. Abby pulled off my shoes and began to rub my feet with all her might.

"No, you aren't going to die; you aren't." Over and over she called my name: "Sue! Sue! Come back! Come back!" Finally I began to breathe normally again. I sat up and rubbed my arms. My skin was as cold as ice and ghastly white.

"I looked death right in the face, Abby. Right smack in the face!" I could see by her face she believed me, but I did feel rather foolish.

A little while later as I walked into the house from work, the phone was ringing. It was my brother Joe calling to say that Mother was dead. I should have felt relief. The last time I'd seen her, her body had shriveled to nothing; her bones looked as though they would burst through her skin; her eyes were vacant. I'd prayed for her to die.

Why was I sobbing? Why was my body shaking, from the bottoms of my feet to the top of my head? Why was there a jarring pain in my skull that felt like a jabbing knife? My mind played connect the dots. *Of course! The cancer has metastasized in my brain,* I thought. *My mother is dead! My mother is dead and her funeral will simply be a rehearsal for my own!*

My family tried to comfort me, but I couldn't be comforted.

That night in bed I relived the experience in the office. I rewound and played it again as if on a tape recorder. I wanted to unlock the mystery. Why did I feel as though I was smothering at the time of Mother's death? Another one of life's inexplicable scenarios. I never slept. I never shut my eyes.

The next day, as we pulled into the parking lot of the big white funeral home in Boca Raton, I wondered if they had sold Mother's casket.

Nine months is a long time to hold one, I thought. We walked into the dimly lit parlor. How beautiful she looked—not sick at all—dressed in the peach-colored chiffon dress I'd bought her so long ago, lying in the peach-lined casket.

That night I sat on Mother's bedroom floor and sorted through her keepsakes. Not much was left. She had already divided the important things among my brothers and me. There were newspaper clippings and her high school yearbook, her wedding book, and beautifully penned obituaries of her mother and grandmother—and pictures. I looked closely at each photograph. Who were these sepia-toned people? I reached for what appeared to be pages torn from an old family Bible, records listing births and baptisms, weddings and deaths. As I noted the dates, I couldn't help wondering what went between. There were no clues. What were their fears? Their disappointments? Their joys? What would *my* descendants know about me?

Mother's funeral was funny. Nothing related to her or her life. The elderly minister centered his message around the story of a yellow dog named Caesar. It wasn't even an interesting story, only that the dog had died and been sadly mourned by his human family. Caesar had been placed in the ground forever.

"If our dear friend did not know Jesus," he motioned

toward Mother's casket, "then her life was in vain, nothing more than this yellow dog named Caesar." I giggled under my breath. Surely one of my brothers would stand and challenge what was being said. Would they let this man get away with it, allow him to drone on and on and never mention our mother or our grief?

"I'll stand up myself. I'll tell him." I would tell him about her deep abiding faith and her special gift of hospitality; how rarely a Sunday meal passed without someone being invited so they wouldn't "have to eat alone."

Didn't he know what an inspiration she had been to us in life . . . and in death? What about our grief and mourning? Did he have no words of comfort to offer? Just as I was poised and ready to stand, I thought, *Of course not! I can't do that, because it isn't really happening! I'm on another of my wild mind trips.*

What happened next brought me back to reality in a hurry. I saw my brothers exchange brief glances and saw Jon give me a knowing look. I could feel my husband's body shudder slightly in laughter. Dear God, I was sane! I *was* sane!

We were able to laugh about Caesar as we followed the hearse into the cemetery. The laughter didn't last long though as the reality of the moment sank in. Mother had joked, "Bury me in Florida and I'll come back to haunt you!" We undoubtedly were in for a double dose of haunting. Jim had insisted on burying her in Florida. *Lantana,* Florida, home of the *National Enquirer!* I didn't know it at the time, but the graves were one on top of the other, bunk-bed style, and Jim would be on top.

At the gravesite I quietly spoke to the old minister, who perhaps had preached too many funerals in a part of the country where folks go to live out their final days and where death is such a common occurrence.

"Please say *something* about our mother," I pleaded. He put aside his notes and did what I had asked.

We stood huddled together, not against cold, but against the unfamiliar tropical air that tasted like salt. I glanced down and saw stubby, coarse grass growing up through sand. Above me were tall stalks of palm trees that flared minimally against a too blue, too clear sky, fine for a resort playground, but not suitable to shade a mother's grave.

My eyes scanned the markers with their unfamiliar names. Why couldn't Mother be buried beside Daddy on that beautiful plot of earth in the West Virginia hills, next to Mae and Elmer and where the family marker was already in place?

Chapter 9

Celebrating Your Faith

"I believe in God the Father almighty, Maker of Heaven
and Earth, And in Jesus Christ His only Son
our Lord . . ."

The Apostles' Creed. We often say it in unison in our
church services. I like repeating it until it rings in my
head like the words to a familiar song. And I like the *exacts* of
it—kind of like my husband telling me about the car.

"Have your car serviced. Do it on a Tuesday when they
aren't busy. Speak directly with the service manager. Take this
list with you so they don't miss anything. Charge it to Visa
and pick it up before 4:30 so you miss the busy time."

Okay! Now that you've explained it, I can handle it. I like
that approach much better than when he mutters, "Car needs
servicing." I can ignore the mutterings for weeks on end.

Before my illness I knew the basics, that I was God's child
and that I would be in Heaven when I died. But beyond that
it was mutterings. Now that death was looming, it seemed
prudent to figure out exactly what it was I could really stake
my life on.

I grew up in a fundamentalist church where repeating the
Apostles' Creed would not have been an acceptable part of
the service. In fact, we steered clear of anything that could be
thought of as *high church*. We felt following an "order" of
service might cause us to fall into a "form" of worship rather
than being led by the Holy Spirit. We were proud that our

money went to missions, not stained glass and steeples. And we had no beautiful edifice because we weren't hung up on bricks and mortar. Perhaps we *were* hung up, though, on not being hung up.

Once I attended a magnificent Episcopal church with my friend Patsy. How I admired the architecture, the stone façade and imposing archways. Afterward I hungered for stained glass, dark polished wood, real pews, and repetitions that seemed to ring with beauty and authority.

My parents' church began in a little Christian bookstore on the mezzanine floor of the old People's Store (later Stone and Thomas) in Charleston, West Virginia. A small group of employees began a Bible study, and as the group grew, they found bigger places to meet—a store front, an automobile showroom, and then a large house, which was gutted and re-modeled to provide Sunday school classrooms and a meeting room. The chairs in the meeting room were nice thick theater seats they found in a salvage store.

"If those seats could talk!" laughed one of my mother's friends.

"We'd get an earful for sure. They've seen some sin in their time, I'd say," answered another. As a child I tried to imagine all the things those chairs might say if they *could* talk.

Eventually we did build a regular church building, not of stone with graceful archways, but of cinder block! Even though it had no steeple or stained glass, I did breathe a sigh of relief that I could finally invite my friends for Bring Your Neighbor Sunday to somewhere besides an automobile show-room.

"God said it, I believe it, and that settles it for me." That seemed to be the answer for everything! Perhaps it really was a pat answer that excused folks from thinking. My church would not have dealt with God's coincidences, like the myste-rious rose petals scattered up the hill at the moment of Dad-dy's death. And our very Christianity would have been in question if we admitted that sometimes our prayers didn't get higher than the ceiling, as they didn't seem to when Mother was sick.

Judgments that I didn't understand were often made. For instance, a couple from church had a car accident Sunday morning. "What can you expect," I heard someone say, "Joe and Gertie went for a drive instead of going to church. That's why they had that wreck!" Obviously, if they had been inside the church building, they wouldn't have wrecked their car, but wasn't the implication that the accident was a form of judgment? I wondered about the dear old lady they called a saint who never missed church in her life but whose house burned to the ground. The inconsistencies were great.

What about the Sunday school superintendent who was considered "godly" and whose wife, on the other hand, was a "real doozy, all that dyed black hair and no zeal for the church." The two of them went on vacation, had a terrible car accident, and she was killed. He recovered and went on to marry someone who had "zeal for the church equal to his own!" Did God do him a favor? I couldn't explain it.

The service itself, most of all the music, was a child's delight. It was unpredictable and fun. Even though we sang songs from the hymnbook, we almost always sang choruses too.

> Deep and wide,
> Deep and wide,
> There's a fountain flowing
> Deep and wide,

we sang. I liked that song because I didn't have to "Sit still, Sue! Sit still, Sue! Sit still!" Everyone did the hand motions, even the old people.

Better yet, I liked the chorus,

> Hallelu-, Hallelu-, Hallelu-, Hallelujah;
> Praise Ye the Lord!

First time through in unison, second time men and boys on the "Hallelu-" and women on the "Praise Ye the Lord." Then it really got exciting! We popped up and sat down in turns. Men up for "Hallelu-" and women for "Praise Ye the

Lord." Up and down. By this time, if things weren't totally out of hand, the song leader would say, "Let's see who can sing the loudest." We kids, at least, would scream our parts at the top of our lungs.

Testimony time was an important part of almost every service, and I could almost predict who would testify. Mr. Plumley would stand up and hop around on his one and only leg and talk about the "saving grace of God," but even at a young age, I knew that anything Mr. Plumley said should be discredited because he chewed tobacco! Without a doubt Jimmy would testify.

Jimmy's story was always the same. Doctors had predicted he would die before he was twelve and here he was eighteen . . . then twenty . . . then twenty-two. Last I heard, Jimmy's still alive, and in his near-sixty years has touched thousands of people with his outgoing personality . . . and Christian testimony! In those days, though, the kids called him crazy and said that someday his oversized head would just explode—pop all over the place. I didn't want to be sitting by him in church when it happened!

Some people talked about a life of sin. I didn't know one thing about a life of sin, but I knew that sometimes it had to do with divorce, and divorce rated right up there with tobacco when it came to sin! It seemed reasonable that God might not like the smell of tobacco. I didn't like it much either. And it seemed reasonable that He didn't like divorce. Even as a child, I knew divorce made people unhappy and divided families and friends. I even thought that possibly God did get bored with a "form" of worship—same old rigmarole, same old prayers, same old words over and over, service after service, week after week. It even made sense that God didn't need stained glass and steeples.

I remember being full of questions when I was a child and even more so as a teenager. For instance, "How do I know the virgin birth of Christ is true?" But even more important to me than whether or not the virgin birth was true— God said it, I believe it, and that settles it—was the issue of wearing makeup. Barn paint, our pastor called it! When I was a young teen two strikingly beautiful women began attending our church. Dramatic hairdos, beautiful clothes, and plenty of makeup. Exactly the way I secretly wanted to look when I grew up.

Things will change now, I thought. *Everyone will see that women are much more beautiful wearing makeup than with color-less faces.*

The church women didn't change, but the two women did. Soon someone set them straight and told them the Lord wanted them to be godly. That meant the Lord couldn't possibly use them until they stopped wearing barn paint and toned down their hair and wardrobes too. They did and in my opinion looked awful! I would have been willing to bet the Lord could have used them just as well wearing makeup, but at my church we didn't bet either!

As I got older I wore makeup. Often, when I was in high school, no one showed up to play the piano for church. When that happened the song leader slipped up to me at the last minute and quietly asked me to go into the restroom and wash off my makeup, so I could play.

Maybe someday I'll be old and "godly" and I'll renounce my lipstick and rouge, I thought, *but for now I'll paint the barn!*

Everyone in that congregation carried a Bible as if it were glued on. Had someone shown up without a Bible, it would have been a more obvious omission than showing up without shoes. And they *used* those Bibles! When the pastor referred to a Scripture reference, I could hear the rustle of pages turning like leaves blowing in the wind.

Everyone, big and small, old and young, was encouraged to *memorize* Scripture. Children were bribed to learn Bible verses with candy, money, and free trips to camp. I won a whole box of Mallow Cup candy bars at camp once, and the thought of it still nauseates me. I ate all of them, one right after another, in the back seat of the church's panel truck, traveling down a winding West Virginia highway.

We not only memorized the verses but we knew the references which we called a "street address." "Genesis 1:1," our teacher would call out, and the first kid to jump out of his seat and begin quoting got a point. The competition became so serious that we held meets with other churches and someone's dad invented an electronic contraption to prove whose bottom left the chair seat first. I loved the excitement, but I doubt I understood the true meaning of those verses. Neither did I know how to apply them to my life—or death.

Years later, as I dealt with cancer, hardly a day went by that I didn't think about dying. It seemed I was always hearing someone make statements such as "He fought a dreadful battle with cancer." *And lost,* I'd add under my breath. I never heard someone say, "He fought a dreadful battle with a ruptured aorta!" How could I not think of my own mortality?

I had embraced the essentials of Christianity and I was sure beyond the shadow of a doubt that when I breathed my last breath I would instantaneously be in heaven. I could quote Scripture to substantiate it. Beyond that, though, there were so many questions, the biggest being "Why?" and followed by, "How can I deal with this on a daily basis between now and dying?"

Physically, I hated losing a body part, but I had a plan for reconstructive surgery. Spiritually I was still looking for answers—not for dying, but for living. Sometimes God sends answers in strange ways. For me they came in the form of an obscure little book. I've heard you can tell how bad your case is by how many books people bring you. Along with flowers, balloons, and fruit baskets, my friends had been sending books at such a pace I'd begun stacking them in a corner. One day a book called *The Healing Power of Christ* arrived from Carolyn, my sister-in-law. Unlike the others, this book had been around a while. It was without a jacket and stained as though someone had handled it with mayonnaise on his fingers. It was dog-eared, and its pages were yellow with time.

"It's old and out of print, and I'd really like to have it back," Carolyn said when she called. "It's something I want to keep. It's meant a great deal to me."

Maybe the only reason I read it was that Carolyn wanted it back. I also knew that she would no doubt call some morning to discuss it. So right away, I leafed through the text with every intention of skimming a little here and a little there, to get ready to bluff my end of the conversation.

"Episcopal Church"—The words on the very first page jumped out at me. There were references to *The Book of Common Prayer,* the sacraments, and the confessions. Instead of Mary and Paul, the author referred to the Virgin Mary and Saint Paul. I could almost smell the dark polished wood of the Episcopalian church in Charleston. I remembered the beauty of the sun shining through the stained glass, the singsongy chant of the priest, the response of the congregation. I was hooked and for all the wrong reasons.

This book instantly became part of my daily routine. I felt compelled to worship God and it appealed to some unexplainable need for beauty and form and organization in that worship. And yet it was something more. I didn't know what.

"Coming to God repeatedly is good," it said. At its urging, I began to repeat the Lord's Prayer often; and for the first time in my life, I found meaning in its words. It became my own at times when I felt my feeble words weren't getting any higher than the ceiling. Likewise, the repetition of the Apostles' Creed caused me to take its message to heart and find comfort in being able to narrow down to the exacts.

Eventually Carolyn and I did have our discussion, and I returned the book to her. Four years later when I was visiting her in California, I asked, "Do you still have that little book you loaned me when I was sick? I miss it."

"I miss it too. I have no idea what happened to it. I loaned it to someone when I was still living in Phoenix, and I don't remember who it was." She explained she'd made several calls trying to track it down.

When I returned to Nashville, my secretary and I called a number of priests, publishers, bookstores, specialists in out-of-print books, and even the Episcopalian Book Club, trying to track down a copy. No luck.

A year later, on the day of my five-year, cancer-free celebration, a package arrived from Carolyn. I tore open the gift wrapping and discovered the well-worn book. Inside the cover Carolyn had lovingly written:

Dearest Sue,

I know you are aware this is more than an old book. It has had a curious odyssey. First, it taught me about healing long before I knew how much I needed it personally; then later, for Webb [her son who was healed from cystic fibrosis]. It traveled through a few other hands and then came into yours. Now it is back to you, a permanent home in celebration of God's great gift to you and to your family who loves you so.

Love,
Carolyn.

This profound book—this special message from God— that had been my spiritual food in the most difficult year of my life was in my hands again. I stretched out on my chaise longue and hoped that no one would interrupt as I opened the pages.

As I'd done five years earlier, I read in no particular order, just grabbing a sentence here and a paragraph there, this time driven by excitement. Nothing jumped from the pages. Nothing at all. Then I started at the beginning, thinking I would read straight through page by page. I found insights and observations worth contemplating, but not at all the kind of stuff I would stake my life on. Not at all what I'd remembered.

Aha! Page 88. This must be it! "Coming to God is repeatedly emphasized throughout the New Testament and especially in the Lord's Prayer. Here we ask, 'Give us this day our daily bread.' We cannot store up God's grace. He wants us to come to Him continually." That had certainly helped me five years earlier.

I remembered how I prayed the Lord's Prayer over and over when I had no words of my own. In the margin, I saw that I'd made a faint pencil mark at the beginning of the sentence. My eyes backtracked to the last line of the paragraph before. ". . . the one who comes to Me I will by no means cast out" (John 6:37). *Hmmm, I learned that as a child,* I thought.

I thumbed on a few pages. "To the precise extent that we trust Him, we are enabled to live in His peace without fear for today or apprehension for the future." Yes! Yes! That helped me so when I awoke with night terrors—those moments that everyone with a life-threatening illness experiences. I practically skipped the next sentence. After all it was just Scripture, and I knew it by heart:

> You will keep him in perfect peace,
> Whose mind is stayed on You,
> Because he trusts in You.

Good grief! I could even remember the street address: Isaiah 26:3!

This book didn't seem worth the reading, much less the effort we had put into finding it. Other than a few choice nuggets, *The Healing Power of Christ* seemed boring, provincial, and not too well written. I picked it up a few times over the next week or so, read a few pages, and put it down again, shaking my head in wonder at what could possibly have made me think it held life's answers.

Like having a string around my finger, but being unable to remember why it was there, the secret of the book gnawed at my mind. Perhaps the intense chemotherapy drugs I had been taking caused me to find meaning when there really was none. Finally it came to me, like the light bulb-over-the-head in the comics, and I ran to get the book.

Page 6: "My grace is sufficient for you, for My strength is made perfect in weakness" (2 Cor. 12:9).

Page 7: "Please let a double portion of your spirit be upon me" (2 Kings 2:9). Oh, how I'd prayed for a double portion. Again on page 7: "They shall possess double; Everlasting joy shall be theirs" (Isa. 61:7).

I turned the pages. "Lo, I am with you always, even to the end of the age" (Matt. 28:20).

On and on, I uncovered truths that were there, not only before Emily Gardiner Neal wrote *The Healing Power of Christ,* but before the very foundation of the earth.

The secret was found at last! The mystery was a mystery no longer. The comfort and peace—the words that had empowered me to face the most overwhelming interference of my life—came from God's Word, faithfully transcribed by Emily Gardiner Neal, because of its application to her own life. The power was in the same Scriptures that I'd been cajoled, bribed, and sometimes badgered to learn as a child in a little fundamentalist church in West Virginia.

I read on with a new eagerness. "For to me, to live is Christ, and to die is gain. . . . For I am hard-pressed between the two" (Phil. 1:21, 23), and then "Today you will be with Me in Paradise" (Luke 23:43).

Five years before, I'd read these pages that spoke of death as the final triumph for the Christian—perhaps the ultimate healing! I'd thought of my daddy then, and I thought about him again now. I remembered the words he spoke on his deathbed: "It's so beautiful!" He was not going to the unknown.

"Today you will be with Me in Paradise." What more does a Christian really need to know?

Chapter 10

The Green Frog of Christmas

More than anything that year I wanted Christmas to be what it usually was at our house: memorable. I was determined to have an eventful, rambunctious Christmas even though the chemical build-up from ten months of chemotherapy left me feeling ugly, puffy, lethargic, and full of poison. I repeatedly had to remind myself to snap out of it!

The doctor juggled the schedule so I could be finished with treatment early in December in the hopes I'd feel good for Christmas. It comforted me to know I had only two months of chemo to go, but I couldn't shake another worry.

One day while waiting for the doctor I'd become restless and looked around for a magazine with which to pass the time. Finding none I picked up my medical file and began to read. Most of it was routine reports detailing my office visits and test results.

Toward the back of the folder I discovered a letter written by my mastectomy surgeon. I read with interest. It said I wasn't a good candidate for reconstructive surgery because I probably wouldn't live that long! After I jumpstarted my pacemaker, my first thought was, *Well, Mister Cowboy Doctor, I've laughed in your face before and I'll do it again. After all, I'm still alive, eleven months later, and I believe I can make it one more month. Maybe longer.* The bravado was skin deep. A lump formed in my throat and a knot settled in the pit of my stomach.

Maybe this is my last Christmas, I worried. I remembered the lyrics to a love song, "If ever I would leave you, it wouldn't be in springtime." The verses that follow say it wouldn't be in fall, winter, or summer either. Maybe I'd write a verse of my own, "If ever I would leave you, it wouldn't be at Christmas. I don't want your second wife to have my manger scene from Bethlehem!"

I thought back over the fun and excitement of Christmases past: the year Wayne gave me a chocolate chess set, the time I gave him a pinball machine. The year I watched two grown men—Wayne and Jon—try to assemble a Barbie condo and never get it right.

One day, several years before, Jon discovered I didn't have a garlic press—powdered garlic was good enough for me—and began to taunt me.

"How can you call yourself a cook? No garlic press?" Then he would turn to whoever happened to be nearby and ask, "Can you believe this woman has no garlic press?"

Long before Christmas that year I knew there would be a garlic press under the tree. The surprise was that it was *electric* or maybe I should say pseudo-electric! Jon had gone to great trouble to attach a thick, long electrical cord, with an industrial-sized plug, to an ordinary garlic press. Had I plugged it in I probably would have been electrocuted on the spot!

Our family loves Christmas! We even love the last-minute shopping, decorating, package wrapping, silver polishing, and baking—the whole family in the kitchen trying recipes, friends stopping by for a few hours with their recipes and going home with a sampling of everything.

"Trr'dition!" we sing, trilling our *Rs* and mimicking the Jewish accents of *Fiddler on the Roof.* Tradition! We certainly have ours. One of our most famous is the traditional Green Frog of Christmas!

Wayne isn't what I'd call a shopper (although he says, "When I die, bury me at the mall . . . so Sue and the girls will visit me often!'"). He loves one store, however, called the Cook's Nook. One year, on one of his trips there, Wayne discovered a plastic ice mold in the shape of a frog. Like a kid with a new toy he bought it and brought it home. Christmas Eve morning he took the ice mold out of the box, filled it with water, added green food coloring, stuck it in the freezer, and checked its progress regularly. "Yeah, it's freezing—the Green Frog of Christmas is freezing nicely," he said.

"We're happy for you, Daddy," Mindy answered in her most *in*-sincere voice and rolled her eyes at the ceiling.

"The Green Frog of Christmas!" Dana and I mouthed the words to each other and held our stomachs and bent over in silent laughter. Wayne was so euphoric he didn't notice our mockery.

Midafternoon on Christmas Eve the celebrating begins at our house. We have a rule: Whoever is spending Christmas must *move in*—for two nights, at least. Most years, once our guests arrive, we can't get rid of them, and the frivolity continues for days, sometimes right up to New Year's. Once we get started, we can't stop: eating, playing games, working jigsaw puzzles, taking naps, watching movies, and then repeating it all, over and over. Dana, Mindy, Jon, Becky, Cara, and Kirby always come, and some years the Nixons—C.B. and Anita, Becky's parents. We're looking forward to having Barry, our new son-in-law, with us next year.

The traditional Green Frog of Christmas was a hit from the first. Wayne waited till everyone gathered for the Christmas Eve festivities: family, friends, and neighbors. Everything was perfect: the smoked salmon with cream cheese and capers, cheese puffs, pâtá and crackers, and a huge array of homemade cookies and candy. When he had everyone's attention, he carried in the exquisite cut-glass punch bowl and placed it on its fancy gilded base. There in the middle of the bright red punch sat the traditional Green Frog of Christmas, glistening proudly. We praised Wayne for his creative idea and workmanship and responded many times to his "Do you like the frog? Huh? Do you like the frog?"

The moment of glory—for both Wayne and the frog—

didn't last long. As the frog began to melt, sounds much like those of a belch—or worse—came forth from his green-ness! Not only that! As the green food coloring blended with the red punch the mixture took on the color of the "or worse," if you know what I mean. We actually only celebrated the *traditional* Green Frog of Christmas once. I suppose it's the retelling of the story that's the tradition!

Each year after our scrumptious buffet, we read the Christmas story from the Living Bible, a paraphrase version we've come to love. Then we share personal thoughts about the true meaning of Christmas, and Wayne leads us in a prayer, thanking God for sending His Son Jesus, who is the true meaning of Christmas.

I'd like to say the spiritual mood lingers, but not so. We're too wound up. We quote "The Night Before Christmas" as best we can, stopping partway through when we remember we've left out something.

"Didn't we forget the part about the obstacle mount to the sky?" someone will say, "and what about the leaves before the wild hurricane fall?" We begin again, but never quite get it right.

Next we pile cookies on a plate for Santa (Christmas morning we find handwritten notes with such bizarre remarks as "Burp!" or "Your cookies made my reindeer sick!"). After everyone is finally in bed, Santa goes to work, making the family room look like a window in a department store, laying the wood for an early morning fire, and getting the big coffee pot ready to plug in.

By five-thirty the next morning (if Wayne can hold off that long), we're all wide-eyed and ready to see what Santa has brought.

It takes several hours to open gifts. We do it one at a time and "ooh and ahhh" over each one. Clothes are modeled on the spot. Then the traditional breakfast: ham slabs cooked on the grill, steeplechase eggs, my chicken-liver-stroganoff, Dana's cheese grits, and Becky's incredible zucchini bread. Later in the day, after naps, Christmas dinner with all the trimmings.

Savoring these wonderful memories made me realize I had no intention of walking off into the sunset to spend Christmas with Elvis! But then again, I thought, this could be my last. A lot can happen in a year.

Something comes over you when you face the possibility of dying. You not only feel a compulsion to get your house in order—throw away the ragged underwear and clean out the drawers—but also there is an overwhelming need to leave something significant behind as a reminder of your life.

For the first time I wrote a Christmas letter, hoping my friends would tuck it away and save it. "Sue's last letter," they would say. I took care not to mention cancer or sickness. After all, I didn't want them say, "Sue's last letter was a real downer. Pitiful . . . just pitiful!" Instead I wrote:

Dear Friends:

As I write this, we're in windy, cold Chicago. Once again, Wayne has kept his promise (made fifteen years ago) that he'd bring me back to do my Christmas shopping and see the sights only a big city can offer.

The snow is blowing wildly, but we are snuggled into our hotel room for the night. What fun we've had eating in our favorite places, enjoying the beauty of North Michigan Avenue with its millions of tiny white lights . . . and shopping . . . special things for the girls gift-wrapped as only Saks can do. A black satin hat for me with a veil down to my chin! Wayne carried the packages and the shopping bags and didn't grumble, not even when I bought the hat . . . only when I wore it!

It's late now, and Wayne is sleeping, but my mind is full of things I want to do this Christmas season . . . fill the cookie jar, light the hill to our house with little white lights like Michigan Avenue, and invite everyone over, especially those I've not seen for a long time. My heart is overflowing with joy, and I'm so very grateful. First of all, for one of God's very best ideas . . . friends! Grateful too for my family! Mindy, who fills my life with fun and little surprises like a love note tucked in my suitcase or flowers by my bed when I wake up. And Dana, who moved into her very own apartment just a couple of miles away but comes home several times a week because she's "homesick." And Wayne, who has given me more love and cherishing than I knew was possible in the almost twenty-five years since he promised to do that.

At this time when "peace on earth" is utmost in our minds, the profundity of Jesus' words rings forth for all time to those who believe: "Peace I leave with you . . . My peace I give you . . . let not your heart be troubled . . . nor let it be fearful."

Love,
Sue

The letter out of the way, I could concentrate on special gifts for my family. Never before had I thought so diligently about what to give. I knew my sympathetic family would understand if I gave them nothing. What a year it had been with the mastectomy, the diagnosis, the aggressive treatment, and Mother's illness and death.

What I really wanted to do was have a pity party, but instead I had a long talk with myself. *Snap out of it!* and *Stop your mullygrubbing!* didn't seem to be working too well. I reminded myself I'd been the center of attention for almost a year. Food had been planned to my liking and schedules arranged for my benefit. My family and friends had become my servants, and everything had revolved around me. Perhaps it was time to reverse roles.

Maybe the reason was selfish—"If this truly is my last year, then I want my family to remember wonderful me"—but whatever my motive, I later realized this was a turning point. I think it would have been easy to stay where I was, with people catering to my whims. I've met several women who have never managed to get beyond this point. One woman told me, "I had cancer twenty-five years ago (which she told me about in great detail), and even though they tell me I'm cured, I just never got over it; my family still has to do everything for me." After that I wrote a little sign and put it on the wall by my desk that said, "Dear God, please spare me from other women's cancer stories." Maybe I could at least

snap part of the way out of it for the Christmas season . . .
maybe mullygrub slightly less.

One day as I was straightening the laundry room I picked
up a ragged old quilt that had been passed down through the
family. As I unfolded it, a flood of memories unfolded with
it—and an idea as well. As usual, I dramatized,

I can see it now, I thought. Someday when one of my
daughters is famous, she'll be asked, "What was your best
Christmas gift ever?" She'll think a moment and answer,
"The last year my mother was with us she had some pieces
from an old quilt framed . . . one for me and one for my
sister . . . and there were two more, I believe, for her brothers." Then she'd tell about the envelope on the back of the
picture frame that tells the story of the quilt. Tears would
come to her eyes and her voice would break: "Such a unique
idea, such a treasure!"

Well, it may not happen as I've described, but the framed
quilt pieces made quite a hit with my family, and there wasn't
a dry eye on Christmas morning as we read the story aloud
together.

CHRISTMAS 1983

My gift to you is a sunflower . . . and a story.

This pattern is called Sunflower, and this tattered piece
was once part of a quilt made by the ladies of the Langsville,
Ohio, Christian Church, where my grandparents attended.
My first memory of it is tracing its pattern as I lay on the
daybed at Grandma Entsminger's. When my grandmother
died, it became my mother's and for years it was folded at
the foot of her bed.

When it became mine, I had no idea of its value or the
sentiments I should have felt. I took it on picnics, used it as
a tablecloth, and spread it on the floor when I rolled around
with my babies. I bleached it and put it through too many
washings until it was worn and falling apart. Still I couldn't
throw it away. The patterns were too beautiful. The tiny,
fine stitches would be hard to find in today's handiwork.
Maybe in this frame, its beauty will last another generation
or two. Here's its story:

When I was a child, I used to spend weeks at a time with Grandpa and Grandma Entsminger at their home in the country near Langsville, Ohio, and later with Aunt Annie and Aunt Maggie a few houses down the road at the "old home place." The home place was built on property given to our ancestors as payment for service in the Spanish-American War. It was a gracious old farmhouse and was used by our large family as a place to come home to. I remember many wonderful reunions there.

Church was important to everyone in the community, and since there was only one, the Christian Church, that's where everyone went (Aunt Maggie always attended but reminded us she was still a Presbyterian since she still held her membership in the Presbyterian church in Zanesville).

I was fascinated by the pump organ in the church and even more so with Clarice, the lady who played it. Clarice had been Mother's friend since they were young girls. She was beauitul, though born crippled—in those days, they called it hunchback—and to me her predicament seemed both tragic and dramatic. I couldn't keep my eyes off her, and when I got home I would hurry to the piano and pretend that I too was crippled!

The church didn't have a minister—at least not regularly—but it did have a choir. Visitors were always asked to sing, and as soon as our family walked in we were ushered up the center aisle past the pot-bellied stove to the choir loft. Daddy would sing at the top of his voice, but I would be more than a little embarrassed.

Quilting day was a monthly occasion, and the ladies arrived early, prepared to spend as many hours as possible. It was held in different homes, but the old home place was a favorite spot because of its large parlor. This was a special time for those farm women, women whose nearest neighbor was miles away, whose shopping experience was limited to the general store in Langsville and the Montgomery Ward Catalog.

There were no television sets in those days, and the telephone party line was for emergencies, not a place to share intimacies. After all, "party line" meant that the whole community could be listening!

The women would set up their quilting frame, drape

their unfinished work across it, take their places around it, and begin a wonderful day of gossiping, laughing, and eating (not all that different from our get-togethers today). As they stitched and chatted, their fingers were busy creating quilt patterns: sunbonnet girls, double wedding rings, butterflies, and sunflowers—beautiful kaleidoscopes of colorful fabric bits that became a work of art. More importantly, for them, a blanket of warmth to keep out the cold of a winter's night.

The busy scene, like a Norman Rockwell painting, is still in my mind; but most of all, I remember impressions of ordinary people creating a masterpiece.

Mrs. Laidley was rather heavy, but that wasn't important in those days. In fact I heard them say that a hefty woman was a good sign her husband was supporting her well. Laurie Folden, my grandma's best friend, was small and fragile looking. Her son was a pilot and once landed his plane in the pasture next to her house. They talked about that for years.

I remember Elsie, whose laughter was loud and boisterous, and I wonder now if her handiwork was a bit less exact than the others' since she was having such a hilariously good time.

Aunt Annie's stitches were probably tight just like she held her needle . . . and her mouth even more so. I could tell from her voice she was often sad and worried about things the others never even thought of. I knew Aunt Annie's story, although she never spoke of it. One morning her young husband had kissed her goodbye and gone outside and shot himself. They found his body by the fence. I never heard an explanation as to why, but in those days children didn't ask questions. No wonder, though, there wasn't as much joy in Aunt Annie's heart as there was in the hearts of her quilting sisters who had loving husbands to cook and bake and do for.

Aunt Maggie had an edge on the others. She'd been to California—her daughter lived there—and she knew first hand what *they* were doing in California. She'd even taken ceramics while she was there and brought back her handiwork. And of course, Aunt Maggie was a Presbyterian.

Barbara, the local beautician didn't make it to quilting day. Maybe that was good because it gave the others a good

chance to discuss the fact that she had divorced her husband
and had bleached her hair to boot! Neither of those things
had been done in Langsville before!

. . . and so, those country women and others who've
faded from my mind worked together making a necessary
household item. To them it probably seemed natural . . .
quite ordinary . . . not at all special. Little did they know as
they pursued their routine, their monthly ritual, that they
were creating a treasure of history for us to enjoy. Had they
known, they probably would have been too embarrassed,
too self-conscious, to work . . . these country women. They
weren't trying to impress or build a name for themselves;
they were just using their God-given talent to do what they
knew to do . . . albeit ever so humble.

Maybe there's a lesson here for us who hold their
memory! All that's left is a sunflower . . . a piece of
history . . . and a story . . .

. . . and that's my gift to you.

While I was planning my last gifts for my family, Wayne
was going through his own dilemma. For years he'd admired a
diamond ring guard that would encase my emerald-cut engagement ring and secretly planned to buy it for me on our
twenty-fifth wedding anniversary, a year and a half away. His
problem was that I might not live that long. After much
thought and consultation with Salem, our jeweler, he decided
I would have my ring guard for Christmas.

A week before Christmas, my daughter noticed that I'd
lost the emerald-cut diamond from my engagement ring, and
though we searched the house over, it was nowhere to be
found. "Like finding a needle in a haystack," I commented
and reminded myself it was insured and it could be replaced.
Wayne wasn't so easily placated. In fact, I'd never seen him so
upset. "Honey, it's okay," I told him. "I can take care of it
after Christmas, when things aren't so busy." He worried
about it constantly and crawled around on his hands and
knees peering under every piece of furniture in the house.

Three days later and four days before Christmas, I was
sitting at the kitchen table with Mary Shillis, our neighbor,

when she jumped to her feet, ran to the corner where we feed the cats, moved their dish aside, and yelled, "I found it. Call Wayne!" Wayne was home in a matter of minutes, grabbed the stone and the ring, and breathlessly exclaimed, "Don't worry. I'll get it fixed for you!"

When I opened my package on Christmas morning there was my old ring surrounded by fourteen sparkling diamonds. I was surprised and Wayne was glowing. Sure, he had some frantic moments, but ultimately his gift was presented in the very best possible way.

I often remind Wayne that I tricked him into buying me the beautiful ring and then fooling him again by being alive for our twenty-fifth anniversary!

Chapter 11

Celebrating Your Friends

It happens to some people in the spring; to others in the fall. It happens to me immediately after Christmas. Each year as I pack away the Christmas decorations, I am consumed by the need to get organized! Even though I had a knot in my stomach, a reminder that a treatment was just around the corner, this year was no different.

I carefully wrapped the glass cookie jars that sit on my kitchen cabinets during the holidays, the toys that line the stairway, the front-door arrangement, the manger scene, and the tree ornaments. *As long as I've gone this far, I may as well organize closets and shelves,* I thought. *Then if I die before next Christmas, at least no one will say I was messy!*

Beginning with the shelves in the garage, I threw away twinkly lights that hadn't lit up for years, much less twinkled. I tossed out rusted cookie tins that looked as if they'd been used in rowdy games of kick-the-can, and out went the pitiful papier-mâché angels that seemed more like street people than heavenly beings.

In the closet under the stairway, I discovered and got rid of nine duffel bags we hadn't used in years. In the family room I found three empty drawers—a direct gift from God—and in the guest room I discovered a treasure! There we have an old French china cabinet that stands with its glass doors swung open to display our *junkories,* a cross between junk and memories. There are museum replicas that Wayne and I brought back from a trip to Greece years ago; interesting containers we chose from the Russian Pavilion gift shop at the Montreal World's Fair; old family pictures in their original cardboard frames; and an assortment of antiques.

From Wayne's side of the family there's a beaten up wooden shoe form, a delicate fringed linen hand towel, and his father's baby shoes. From my side, there's a tiny gilded French mirror, a small cheese basket, a minaudière evening purse, and two well-worn autograph books that had belonged to my grandparents, Lewis and Carrie Entsminger.

I reached for one of them and examined the beautifully tooled leatherwork. Slivers of aged, brownish paper flaked into my hands and floated to the carpet like a lazy snowfall. It was curious that this book had been in my possession for years and yet I'd never looked at it.

What words of wisdom might Grandma's friends have to offer, I wondered, and I opened the book. I moved to sit on the bed and sank back into the pillows, noting the date on the very first page. How ironic that a hundred years to the *exact* day had passed since that entry. A shiver went through me, as sometimes happens when such a strange coincidence takes place. It was as though it were preplanned, inevitable, that I would pick up *that* book on *that* day.

> Carrie, Each autograph the signet be,
> Of some true-hearted friend . . .
> The memory of whose genial soul,
> Will ever sunshine lend.
> May your life be calm and peaceful,
> Gentle as the flowing stream,
> And your life be no more painful,
> Than waking from a dream.
> Friend Carrie, We should live for those
>   who love us,
> Whose hearts are kind and true;
> For heaven that smiles above us,
> And the good that we can do.

Katie Maloy, Amanda L. Snyder, and the others, Grandma's friends, penned such lovely sentiments. I couldn't help but think of my lyricist-poet friend Gloria who can create a beautiful thought or poem or song—words that make me ask, *Why didn't I think of that?* I remembered all the times during my illness that she wrote to me from her travels around the country, and how each message was exactly what I needed at the time.

Most of the cards I received were store bought. Though written by someone at Hallmark, they had the perfect sentiment. Donna and Murray sent a card every week for the entire year I was taking chemotherapy. Sometimes they were fat-little-cherub-and-cabbage-rose effusive, but more often than not, they were grab-your-stomach-and-bend-double funny!

Apparently Grandma too, had friends who preferred silliness over sentimentality.

> May your life be as long,
> as old cheese is strong.
> And as free from care,
> as a baby's head is of hair.
> (Signed) Your friend Abe.

> O! how *mean* you are;
> I wish *I* had some chestnuts, don't you *rats,*
> Yours for fun, J. W. Dietz

Mean? Chestnuts? Rats? Who knows the meaning of those words? My guess is that J. W. and Carrie must've been the best of friends to have a language all their own.

Like Grandma's friends, my friends and I have a private language. Say the word *pantyhose* to Evelyn, she'll roll her eyes, and we'll all laugh, remembering the time at a party when she discovered an extra pair inside her pant leg. Say *earrings* in Lynn's presence, and she'll give you a knowing look that says, *Don't you dare tell that story!* We are such good friends we can communicate with a word or a knowing glance.

My friends and I don't even have to say, *I shouldn't say*

this, but . . . , before we gossip. To me, that's real friendship! And we have slumber parties, regular old junior high school sleepovers! "Wayne's out of town," I'll say. "So's Bob," Joy will answer. "Let's have a slumber party." The group can include Gloria, Peggy, Carlana, Marty, Lynn, or Evelyn—whoever can make it. The more, the merrier!

Once in a while we manage a vacation to the Cayman Islands or a sailing trip on Joy's boat. One of us will mention there's a cheap flight available to Miami where the boat is docked, and the words "I'm broke!" suddenly become "I'll find the money somewhere!"

The boat is the most restful, rejuvenating vacation spot imaginable. There's a captain who worries about where we are going, watches out for storms, and understands the workings of the motor. All we have to think about is whether we have enough suntan lotion and candy bars to make it to the next port.

We call it a working vacation. It's the perfect place to work on a book or script, plan a speech, or write music. Joy has authored forty-five children's books, and Peggy is a writer and inspirational speaker, so they always have works in progress. Lynn, who writes anthems, octavos for choirs, and children's musicals, brings along a keyboard and can whip out a complete musical during a week-long trip. It's not unusual for the rest of us to have to act as a makeshift choir to try out the parts (soprano, alto, tenor, *and* bass) to see if they work.

We spend the first three or four hours of each day working alone; then we discuss our projects together and offer each other advice as we soak up the sun. Afternoons are spent sailing, snorkeling, fishing, or doing nothing.

The best moments of the day are nature's shows. Under sail, we are often joined by porpoise, who think it's great fun to show off, gliding under the boat and up on the other side, high in the air, and back into the water, all the while smiling their gigantic smiles.

Just before sunset we anchor and sit back in our chairs for the show of the day, sunset! We're never disappointed. One of us will undoubtedly break into song, which leads to another and another. Our harmony is clear and perfect, a skill we've never quite been able to recapture on dry land.

After dark we go below for a scrumptious meal, taking our time, and savoring every bite—and savoring our stories, tales not only of our past adventures together, but also husband and children stories. And on occasion old boyfriend stories. Do we want to hear, once again, about Lynn's old boyfriend? . . . and my old boyfriend? . . . and Joy's friend who became a breast doctor? Is there a *National Enquirer?*

Our stories become more interesting each time they are told. We've given each other permission to exaggerate. The flying roach that attacked Marty and me one night in Cayman has grown to man-eating proportions; and we tell about the night Peggy put the wrong kind of soap in the dishwasher, causing it to overflow, as though it were the highlight of our vacation! Another time in Cayman, during a torrential nor'wester, we performed a song and dance routine from *Singing in the Rain,* complete with plastic garbage-bag costumes. In the retelling, the performance now equals an opening night on Broadway.

Friendship, I believe, is built on history, and the telling and retelling of that history cements the friendship.

If we've told it once, we've told it a hundred times, the one about Peggy's favorite jacket that I took to the resale shop by mistake and the owner telling me that nobody in their right mind would buy such an ugly jacket, even in a resale shop.

We know well the saga of Lynn at the Miss Alabama beauty pageant when she forgot her escort, and we laugh our heads off when we recall the time we all went to Houston for a musical. Lynn insisted someone in the next hotel room was being killed, when actually the screams were those of passion.

"You know what Bob always said." Yes, Peggy, we know, but if you repeat it we'll laugh. "He said I took up knitting so I'd have something to *think* about when I talked!" We laugh as though we've never heard it before!

Our ladies-only vacations may seem strange to some people, but we have no problem at all taking off without our husbands. These trips offer a different kind of relaxation from those with our husbands. For instance, you don't hand a man a Spam on white bread! Men want real meals, and they want them when they want them.

"Have we made reservations?" If the answer is yes, then it's, "Why so late?" or just as likely, "Why so early?"

"What kind of place is it? Is it good?"

"Well, gee, I don't know. It says here in the travel guide, it's *bad!* Last tourists who ate there died of ptomaine poisoning!"

Then there's the matter of switching on the TV everytime you walk in the room, which women don't do! And I won't get into the fact that women just kind of mosey off to bed when they feel so inclined, while men say, "Time to go to bed." If we ignore them, they'll say it a little louder: "Time to go to bed!" And if we still ignore them, they'll repeat it, adding, "I'm tired. Aren't *you* tired?"

Before one of our trips we are the epitome of *wifeliness,* with a lot of *let-me-cook-your-favorite-meal-sweetheart,* and *let's-just-spend-the-evening-watching-one-of-those-exciting-football-games-on-TV-baby-honey* talk.

Many times our women-only trips start out as husband trips. It's just that men have such a hard time coordinating their schedules. It seems that when Wayne can go, Bob is busy, and vice versa; when Wayne and Bob manage to work it out, Bill is off someplace wheeling and dealing.

When we do manage to arrange a couple vacation, we love it. It can't be beat for fun and excitement. We pack in enough adventure to last a long time. I love sitting down with my photo albums and reliving those trips: Paul at Ed Debevic's in Chicago in that silly paper hat; the usually quiet Tommy dancing a jig in Greektown; Shillises and Zimbelmans at Diana's, our favorite restaurant.

One whole album has nothing but fishing pictures: Wayne helping Phyllis and Rhonda hold up their king salmon; Bob posing with his rainbow trout as though he had fished all his life; and Paul looking like an ad for *Sporting Man* magazine.

Before my mastectomy, year of therapy, and reconstructive surgery, things like this didn't matter that much. Let's face it, I wasn't the world's most caring, nurturing, *do-unto-others, love-your-neighbor-as-yourself* kind of person—although I would feed someone's cat if asked.

For a while after my mastectomy and the resulting bad news, I preferred to *observe* life, rather than to *participate* in it. I watched people come and go; I saw them talk, laugh, and touch; and I simply wanted to watch. It was as though I wondered what life would be like without me.

Eventually, I moved through that stage and on to a level of participation I never before knew was possible. I didn't want to miss anything! In fact, all of the trips—the slumber parties, photo albums, and journals—have been *since* my cancer surgery. Suddenly I had a new zest for living, and because friendship (with both men and women, and even with my own family) was such an integral part of living, I began evaluating what it meant to be a friend.

An important thing I learned was that people can do only what people can do! Had I realized this before, I would have spent less time being judgmental, asking, *Why didn't he do this?* or *Why didn't she do that?* There were people who seemed glib in regard to my illness, ready with an easy answer. Others made me feel as though what I was going through was worse than it actually was. Some even treated me as though I were dying. That was difficult for me, but as time passed, I began to realize that each person sees things from his or her own personal perspective.

I've always loved to read biographies, especially about political figures. I'll read anything and everything about the Kennedys, short of the *National Enquirer* (and I'll do that in a supermarket line, if push comes to *shove!*). When I see "Kennedy gives birth to two-headed baby," I don't even look over my shoulder to see if the pastor is behind me; I just grab and read!

One of my favorite examples of personal perspective is from a Jackie Kennedy biography in which Lyndon Johnson was making an effort at friendship with Jackie after Jack's death. He sent her flowers, invited her over, and even offered her positions in his administration. On one occasion, he called her *sweetheart* and gave her orders to get on over to the White House and start living again. She was so infuriated, both about being called *sweetheart* and about his condescending attitude, that she referred to him as an oversized cow-punching oaf!

When told that Jackie was upset, Johnson answered, "Where I come from, we call the ladies sweetheart, and the ladies call their gentlemen honey. I've bent over backwards for that woman. I've done cartwheels and deep-knee squats, and all I get is criticism."

Lyndon Johnson was just Lyndon Johnson *being* Lyndon Johnson, with his own set of baggage that came from Texas roots, and Jackie was Jackie, whose feelings were conditioned by her refined progenitors.

In a time of life crises, people are especially vulnerable to the seeming insensitivity of another person's perspective. An author, writing about her mother's illness, tells of a minister who drove six hundred miles to see her mother, but didn't do what they'd expected—didn't offer the comfort they'd hoped for. Does the six-hundred-mile drive count for nothing?

A secretary friend of mine got a call from her boss who'd been in the hospital for a couple of weeks. "Bring your notebook when you come today," he ordered. When she arrived, he began to dictate a list of names. She assumed these were people to whom he'd be sending thank you notes. Instead, he was listing the people he *hadn't* heard from.

"They've hurt my feelings, and I want to make sure I ignore them when they get sick!" he explained.

If I had to reduce this chapter to only one thought, it would be to encourage a person to accept the deep-knee squats; to list the "been theres" instead of the "not been theres," and to gather up the gifts people offer, one by one, and put them in a big basket (figuratively speaking, of course). You'll find the gifts that are brought have a marvelous variety of intangible, immutable qualities, such as humor, joy, acceptance, good conversation, touching, crying, listening, surprise, prayer, and—perhaps the greatest gift of all—time. That source will provide everything you need to get through an illness—or through life, for that matter! So reach in the basket and take what you need as you need it. Use it! Savor it! If there's anything left, pass it on, and for heaven's sake, don't expect everyone's gift to be the same.

Peggy kissed me on the lips during my illness (still does), and her gift to me was that she wasn't worried about catching the plague. Some people turned away from me, or covered their mouths when they stood close to me.

Joy, who we tease about carrying Lysol in her purse to decontaminate toilet seats, could never kiss me, then or now! But Joy knows how to celebrate! She could celebrate a dead dog! She gave me the gift of celebration at every step of the mastectomy, chemotherapy, and reconstructive surgery.

"Another thing behind us," Joy would say as she came up with a new way to celebrate; a box lunch at the office with animal crackers for dessert; a children's book she'd read aloud to me with all the sound effects, much as you would read to a child; parties of all varieties; and the grand finale, a trip to the Grand Cayman Islands.

Joe Shillis, our neighbor, wouldn't think to plan a trip to an exotic island, and Joe doesn't know how to plan parties. He would probably think some of Joy's shenanigans downright silly. He would know how to do other things that lift the spirit. He knows whether the funny noise my car is making is serious or not; if I should cover my plants because of frost; whether there is too much wind to fish; and knows how to cry with me. How rare in a man! Joe came to the hospital, took my hands in his rough ones, and looked into my eyes, and our tears poured. Alice, Joe's wife, was my first visitor each day, having made a stop at church to light a candle signifying her prayers for me.

I didn't know Locher very well at all, so it was a complete surprise when he visited me in the hospital. From my bed I could see a tall, lanky figure pacing back and forth in the hall as though undecided about coming in. It took me a moment to recognize this well-dressed man in a three-piece gray suit. Before I'd only seen him in his white work shirt that said "Locher Bibb" on his left pocket, just beneath "J. B. Cook Auto Parts."

I motioned him in, and after a brief greeting, Locher sat down close to me, put his head in his hands, and said, "My first wife died of that!" I was taken aback, to say the least, but when I looked in his eyes, I knew that what he was really saying was, "I understand."

Many of my male friends were uncomfortable with the fact I'd lost a breast. They were uncomfortable with the *B* word, and they would look at the ceiling, with an occasional hope-I-don't-get-caught glance you know where.

I had two friends—Chris, a young businessman, and Michael, an artist who visited me almost every day. They thought nothing of climbing up on the bed with me, as though it were a slumber party.

"With those legs, who needs breasts?" was one of Chris's lines, and I can't repeat Michael's comment when he arrived with a dozen balloons.

There are those who would criticize the ribald humor of my guests, but the bantering and teasing made up one of my best gifts. It did a great deal for my self-esteem and my ability to think of myself as a normal woman.

Some friends didn't come to visit me in the hospital, but later showed up at my house with a casserole. The gift of casserole is one of the most important! Sometimes I threaten to get sick, just to get some of Kate's lasagna, Alice's potato salad, or Evelyn's soup. Our church members do a remarkable job of caring for families in crises. They're good at feeding both body and soul.

During my illness, I discovered another whole circle of friends I didn't know existed, every-day-of-the-week people. Before, I was too busy for small talk, and I was missing a whole chunk of life that I now hold dear. These every-day-of-the-week people are the folk who pass through my life coincidentally, just because we are in the same place at the same time. As these people saw my vulnerability during the year I was in treatment, they questioned me with concern. Many asked if there was anything they could do. Some told me of their prayers for me.

I could easily have gone the rest of my life, having lunch at Arnold's Country Kitchen, without saying much more than the words, "Meatloaf, mashed potatoes, fried apples, and greens." Jack Arnold could just as easily have filled my plate, pushed his cash register buttons, and taken my money. Now we make it an event.

"Sue Buchanan's here," he'll announce to everybody in the restaurant. Everybody can include country singers, advertising agency people, a former governor, and bums right off the street. "I gotta joke for you."

"What, no seats? Throw somebody out; I need a table." I say at the top of my lungs and laugh at his joke as I go through the line to get my food. One of my proudest moments was when Jack featured my photography exhibit on the slightly greasy plastic-paneled walls of his down-home eating establishment. If I had a choice of showing off my work at Arnold's Country Kitchen or the National Gallery, it would be Arnold's in a New York minute.

I could go to Dillard's Department Store, buy my stockings and eyebrow pencil, check out the shoes, and get home twice as fast if I didn't stop to talk to Gloria. She has been selling me Shalimar since it was eight dollars a bottle and since Dillard's was Cain Sloan. She cared that I was sick, and to this day, she never fails to ask whether I'm still okay.

"How are those little boogers doing?" the woman at the discount bread store asked me the other day.

"They were there the other night at five-fifteen, before it was even dark. Can you believe that? And the one we called Ricky is now Rhonda, because she had three babies," I explain as I pay for my day-old bread and hurry home to feed my raccoons.

The people at Stevens Drug Store—Mrs. Wolf, Ruth, and Dr. Stevens—expect me to stop by to say hello even when I have no prescriptions to fill. When Mrs. Wolf had breast cancer, I visited her at home because she wanted me to come.

The gifts in my basket come not only from my close personal friends, and acquaintances, but also from my every-day-of-the-week friends. Often one of these people says the exact word of encouragement I need for the day.

The basket philosophy of friendship gives me incredible resources, but that's only half of the story. The other half is that I now have the responsibility and privilege of filling baskets myself, and it is by far one of the most rewarding life experiences I have ever known—even when I'm sick and don't feel like it!

Chapter *12*

If It's Broken, Fix It!

That night in the hospital when Dr. Maxwell told me about reconstructive surgery, I knew immediately I would choose that course of action, assuming, of course, I had to have a mastectomy.

Even though I knew nothing about reconstructive breast surgery at the time, I wasn't ignorant about plastic surgery. I knew about it almost firsthand! This may sound like gossip, and I can't mention names, but some of my best friends have had it. There's rhinoplasty (care to guess the derivation of that word?) to correct noses that aren't just right, and there's blepharoplasty for eyes that are puffy and have lost their lid definition, and there's liposuction to slurp away those little blobs of fat that make your clothes fit funny.

Occasionally whole faces must be lifted! My husband has observed that a certain country music star has had her face lifted so much she doesn't have to bend over to pull up her socks—she simply raises her eyebrows! When certain things droop they must be propped up! Need I say more?

Almost everyone I know who has had plastic surgery talks about it openly. Not everyone likes to make jokes about it. I learned that the hard way. My actions, I would like to point out, were egged on by my friends. It seems that they would have counseled me to be more tactful. On the other hand, had they, I probably would have done what I did anyway. Maybe I should have listened to Wayne, who pointed out that if you have to check with other people, then you probably shouldn't do it.

It happened this way. A young business associate of mine, who will go unnamed, didn't try to keep her plans for plastic surgery a secret. She kept us posted each step of the way. She called it by its correct name, rhinoplasty; we called it a "nose job." She told us that she had been shown pictures of various nose structures and with her doctor's help, she'd chosen the one that was best suited for her face. She explained that there were claustrophobic after-effects that would probably cause her to feel panicked and disoriented for a few days, but that she had thought of a way to counter them. She would pack her nose *before* the surgery and get used to it *ahead of time*. Such discipline!

The operation went as scheduled, and I wracked my brain to think of some clever way to cheer her up and help her celebrate her new nose. After all, that's what our group of friends does when one of us is in the hospital. Bob still has the antique bedpan full of cactus we brought him eight years ago when he had his heart attack; and if I live to be a hundred, I'll never forget the seafood buffet with all the trimmings Dan and Phyllis had delivered to my hospital room the night before my reconstructive surgery, or the cake Joy and Minnie brought. It was made to look like the torso—neck to thigh—of a large-breasted woman in a bikini. Every nurse, doctor, and ambulatory patient on the floor, as well as my dignified Presbyterian pastor, ended up in my room for a piece of cake before the evening was over.

My idea for cheering up my friend who was having rhinoplasty wasn't *that* bold. I thought it was a good idea. First of all, I baked a cake—a scratch cake—and in retrospect I can see that I should have simply delivered the cake, expressed my good wishes, and left. It was the homemade get well card that caused the problem.

"Choose which nose you would prefer." I printed in bold letters on the front.

"A funny one?" it said on page two, where I pasted a picture of Mickey Mouse.

"A famous one?" it said beside Jacqueline Kennedy's photo.

"A political one?" beside Richard Nixon's mug.

There were other pictures and other blurbs, but you get the idea! The punch line, I'm sure you've already guessed: "Now that you've picked your nose, wash your hands and have some cake." I signed my name and set out to deliver the cake, chuckling all the way.

By the time I handed over my prize, I was smiling my toothiest smile. I couldn't wait for my friend to read the card. I waited for a reaction. I'm still waiting. She apparently saw no humor in it. No humor at all. I wasn't invited to stay for tea. I wasn't thanked. I didn't see her for days, and when I did, she was cool and didn't mention my card. To this day, every time I see her beautiful profile, I wonder how I could have missed so completely.

So the card was tasteless. Sometimes *life* is tasteless!

Ah yes, "there is some myth for every man [and woman] if we but knew, it would make us understand all that he [she] did and thought." I didn't say that; Yeats did. However, I've pondered the concept more than once. I don't know why one woman would choose plastic surgery and another wouldn't anymore than I know why years ago, when we lived on Sixth Street, our neighbor Simon Jones had such a fit when I cut his daughter Simona's never-been-touched-by-scissors hair.

Even then aesthetics were important to me, and I knew at that tender age, Simona's haircut made her look 100 percent better! I thought the whole neighborhood would thank me, but when my mother hung up the phone, she asked in her most incredulous tone of voice: "Sue, did you cut Simona's hair?" and before I could answer—and certainly before thinking to thank me—she turned to my father and said: "That was Simon Jones. Sue cut Simona's hair, and Simon is hoppin' mad!"

Now that I think of it, no one ever *did* thank me! That's twice!

Even as a child I was apparently vain. At the age of three I was in a fashion show at the People's Store. I did just as I was told until I got to the end of the runway. There I remained despite backstage whispers that got louder and louder: "Pst! Sue, come back now. Sue . . . Sue . . . *Suzanne!*"

Loving the attention, I kept parading around, adding bows and spins that weren't rehearsed until an embarrassed fashion director came to pull me out of the spotlight—but not before I caught sight of our neighbor, held the back of my skirt high above my head, gave a three-hundred-and-sixty-degree spin that revealed my underwear, and yelled, "Oh, Clurey (short for Mrs. McClure), isn't this the pwettiest dwess you ever laid eyes on?"

Not long after, of course, I became Mrs. Vandertweezers, dressed in that satin blouse—a discard from Aunt Ginny—that came down to my ankles, and a hat out to there. I wore her old shoes that let my painted—when my mother would let me paint them—toes poke out, and around my neck was an animal that bit its own tail. Underneath all this I pinned my daddy's socks for bosoms.

Mrs. Vandertweezers grew up to love flashy clothes right down to her underwear. Even there she much preferred lizard skin over plain cotton, trimmed in little animal parts if possible! An exaggeration of course, but the truth is Mrs. Vandertweezers still lived inside me, and the lady had no intentions of filling her bra with rolled-up socks for the rest of her life! Reconstructive surgery was the only way to go.

Not long ago, I asked Dr. Maxwell's office for my medical file to jog my memory as to the specifics of my reconstructive surgery. The first thing I noticed when I opened the file was a letter. I had written it the week of my biopsy.

Dear Pat,
    You were the only ray of hope in a week filled with bad news. Thank you for being there.
    In the past two or three weeks it amazes me how many women have shared with me that they have had my same experience! It blows my mind that rarely do I find someone

who has known her options—especially that she doesn't have to live her life deformed.

Thank you for loaning me the book. Hold a place for me in your busy schedule for a year from now—February or March—and then watch out! I have a lot of living to do!

Sincerely,
Sue Buchanan

The next thing that captured my attention was twenty-two pages of information about Dr. Maxwell. I had asked his receptionist to include his bio when she sent my file. As I thumbed through his impressive list of accomplishments, it occurred to me that this was a first. I'd never been given—nor had I thought to ask for—this kind of information before.

It wouldn't be such a bad idea to put this on the list of things to ask for when doctor shopping, I thought.

There was correspondence to Pat from Cowboy Doctor along with my operative records and pathology reports for both surgeries. His preoperative notes for the lumpectomy were easy to decipher.

I first examined this 45-year-old white female on 1/14/83 as a referral from Dr. Patrick Maxwell. (This is incorrect. The referral came from Dr. Tipton.) The patient complained of a mass deep in the left breast which she had detected herself. She was particularly concerned because her mother had had carcinoma of the breast and she had recently had a friend die of carcinoma of the breast. On examination, the patient was found to have huge symmetrical breasts. At the 6 o'clock position half way between the central portion of the breast and its periphery deep in the breast, was a somewhat movable, well delineated, slightly irregular, 2 cm. mass. No axillary nodes were palpable. No other dominant masses were felt. In the office, I attempted to decompress the lesion by aspiration. The lesion could not be decompressed. Subsequently, a mammogram was obtained. The mammogram suggested that the lesion was likely malignant. Biopsy was advised. The patient requested that no procedure other than biopsy be carried out. She had not been able to bring herself to accept a mastectomy. The patient was thus admitted to the hospital for excisional biopsy.

Did I detect a note of sarcasm in those words? "The patient couldn't *bring* herself to accept a mastectomy." Not true! The patient suddenly realized she had options.
The pathology report was scary.

The approximate center of the specimen has an unencapsulated, circumscribed, fleshy, gray nodule, measuring 1.6 cm. in diameter. Frozen section diagnosis is infiltrating duct carcinoma . . . control is submitted in cassette FS-1 and representative selected sections are submitted in cassettes A, B and C. Tumor cells have large moderately plemorphic vesicular nuclei with prominent nucleoli and vacuolated cytoplasm.

That's just a portion of it, and only for the lumpectomy. The report on the mastectomy is too frightening for words!
The next piece of correspondence is to my oncologist from Dr. Maxwell. It speaks of my "guarded prognosis" and says that after discussing the various techniques of breast reconstruction, I "tentatively selected to undergo transverse rectus abdominus myocutaneous flap reconstruction of the left breast with the combined abdominal reconstruction (lipectomy)." That meant he would be making my new breast out of my stomach fat, but of course he couldn't afford to say it so simply; after all he had twenty-two pages of credentials!
The letter also discussed whether or not it would be a good idea at the time of reconstruction to remove the right breast due to the high probability of cancer's recurring there. There are no further notes on this, but I remember that my oncologist recommended this precaution. The final paragraph says, "I wish her prognosis were better, as she certainly could give a ray of hope to many women who have breast cancer."
I remembered the fears. I also remembered the excitement when I knew at last that reconstructive surgery would be a reality. Finally I would be having my body fixed. For a year, I'd avoided undressing in front of my husband, chosen dresses with high necklines, and stayed clear of mirrors.

Getting up in the night to go to the bathroom was a nightmare in itself. Without my prosthesis my balance was off, and I would fall flat or at best stumble into the furniture. I was one big bruise waiting to happen. When I was dressed and had the weighty prosthesis in place, I was once again in balance.

I cringed at the thought of wearing a bathing suit. Before Wayne and I went to Puerto Rico, I bought one designed specifically for mastectomy patients. It had a high neckline but not high enough. When it was wet it drooped, and I was always pulling at it for fear it would reveal my concave chest. When I went for a dip, I would lay a cover-up by the side of the pool so I could quickly put it on the minute I came up out of the water.

The other time I got an overdose of the hated bathing suit was when Joy took me to the Grand Cayman Islands as a reward for making it to the end of chemo and still being alive. There we wore our swimsuits all day every day, only dressing at night for dinner.

Knowing I'd be having reconstructive surgery as soon as I got back to Nashville helped, as every day I put on the baglady-baggy, dingy suit and self-consciously began my day. The first thing I was going to do when I got my body back was burn the ugly bathing suit. Then I'd buy a new one—a *pink* one!

A couple of months ago I mentioned to my friend Rose Miller at The Institute for Aesthetic and Reconstructive Surgery at Baptist Hospital that I was trying to remember the details of my reconstructive surgery.

"Why don't you watch a surgery? Dr. Maxwell wouldn't mind." I loved the idea, and before I knew it, she had arranged it. I'd be observing a double mastectomy and reconstructive surgery that would use the patient's stomach tissue to form both new breasts. The woman didn't have cancer, but was plagued with suspicious lumps and a family history that put her at high risk. She was one of many women choosing prophylactic mastectomy as breast cancer prevention.

The day of surgery finally arrived, and after I'd donned

my scrubs, complete with hat, footies, and mask, I was invited to meet the patient. She was "happy" with medication and greeted me cheerfully and introduced me to her husband. Our mutual doctor explained to her why I was there, that I had experienced similar surgery and was writing a book to help other women. We had immediate rapport. (In her drugged state she'd have had rapport with a chimpanzee!)

"I saw your picture and note in Dr. Maxwell's book," she chuckled, and I knew she was referring to the snapshot of me in my pink bathing suit along with the note to Pat that said, "Thanks to you, women with remarkable bodies are sleazing the beaches of the world."

We chatted until the gurney pushers came to take her the short distance to the operating room.

As I walked out, her husband took her in his arms for a last embrace against what I observed as lush, full breasts. I wondered if they'd made love the night before and if she had sobbed silently in the night as I'd done before my mastectomy. I remembered my own doubts and my wondering if the same intimacy could ever again be achieved.

I walked through the doors with all the warning signs. The I-don't-want-to-know-what-goes-on-beyond-there double doors. I'd been in operating rooms dozens of times before for filming purposes. Usually one of the nurses volunteered to be the "patient," and we simulated the scene for benefit of the camera.

I glanced at the digital clock on the wall: 7:30.31. *Today it's for real,* I thought as I seated myself on a stool against the wall, six or seven feet from the operating table. *I'll get used to it gradually, and as I do I can move closer.* It occurred to me I didn't want to embarrass myself by passing out at the sight of blood.

Not too surprisingly, the things that bothered me most were the odors: floor cleaner, antiseptic, bandages, iodine—the many things that combine to make up the hospital smell. It was overwhelming, and I wondered if I would last through the preliminaries.

I've always been affected by smells, whether it's floor cleaner, dry cleaning fluid, gasoline, or the scent wafting through Marshall Field's dressing room from the lady with the stinky armpits who was there before me. Even the room spray they use to cover the smells gags me. Blended together it becomes Stinky Lady Lemon, or Your Grandfather's Feet Eucalyptus.

It didn't take long to forget myself and be drawn into what was happening in the room. Like the players on a basketball team, the five members of this surgical team prepared for the "game," and for the next five hours I watched them move as one well-oiled machine to accomplish one of the most incredible feats I've ever witnessed.

"Ready for some music?" one of the blue-clad women asked as she pushed a cassette into a player. Windham Hills-type music began to play. The patient chatted easily with the anesthesiologist. As the drugs dripped, dripped, dripped through the I-V and into her arm, her words slowed until they were garbled, then incoherent, and finally nonexistent.

I remember the feeling well. For me it was as though I was traveling down a long tunnel, like the inside of a giant Slinky, toward the darkness of outer space.

How can anyone sleep in that light? The operating room was so bright it seemed to me like an overexposure, with light reflecting harshly off of the many stainless steel surfaces. Four giant octopus-like fixtures overhead could be moved back and forth to shine even more light on the working area. There must have been two hundred instruments: scissors, scalpels, and needles of every size and shape, plus wicked looking implements I couldn't identify.

The surgical staff wore unfashionable garb of green and blue that covered them from head to toe. Only their eyes were visible between mask and cap. No words were spoken. No time was wasted. Everyone had tasks to perform as the patient was readied for surgery.

Her head and outstretched arms were covered with green sheets, and tight elastic stockings were pulled over her feet and onto her legs. They used gigantic needles, perhaps filled with a novocaine-like substance, to puncture her abdomen, her stomach, her breasts. Her body became a rag doll, not feeling a thing. Buttons were pushed on the operating table to reposition her body almost to a sitting position and pictures were taken. The time on the digital wall clock said 7:54.01.

On the patient's body, Dr. Maxwell mapped his plan with a big black felt marker. He drew generous, misshapen *lips* beginning above the navel and extending to the pubic hairline. Everyone relaxed as though they understood there was no damage done if the pen slipped. He continued his markings, having moved to the breast area but he was between me and the patient and was blocking my view.

"Hattie is having surgery next week. I can't imagine having you guys operate on me," said the male assistant. "If I've ever offended anybody in this room, I want you to know I'm sorry! I'd hate to think you were mad at me when you cut me open." Everyone laughed.

Pat stepped back and put the lid on his marker. Automatically three members of the team began swabbing the patient with great quantities of iodine. The smell was strong. They chatted about ordinary things: a Christmas party, a new baby, and midlife crises.

"Mine is almost over. I'm just about out of my Harley-Davidson stage." I couldn't tell if the anesthesiologist was actually into motorcycles, or if the statement was for my benefit. He had a twinkle in his eyes—eyes that quickly glanced in my direction and back again to the panel of lights and gauges before him. Suddenly everyone was aware of my presence. Pat bent to allow one of the nurses to place a steel halo on his head that held an intense direct light.

"She's my circulator," he said, gesturing to the nurse. "She anticipates my needs throughout the surgery. Problem is, when I get home at night I don't have a circulator! Kathy [his wife] refuses!" We laughed.

"Ask questions. Move closer. Feel free to walk around. We'll tell you if you get in our way." I *would* have walked around if they hadn't been about to cut. I lay my pad and pencil in my lap and hung on to my seat with both hands.

It became quiet as incisions were made, first the abdomen and then the breasts. I watched as the black lines became oozy with blood as the scalpel followed the drawn patterns. I was surprised. It was not all that gruesome. I leaned forward to get a better look. Once again each person had a set of chores, all moving together, communicating with a word or a gesture, sometimes with a look. Dr. Maxwell's sure hands worked quickly and expertly, occasionally signaling for an adjustment of the light on his brow or to the operating table.

8:23.12—a breast was placed into a blue napkin. I didn't remember getting up, but I was standing. Windham Hills had been replaced by soft jazz.

9.50.22—breast number two went into a blue napkin, and I watched the surgical assistant trim slivers from it just as he had the other one. The two specimens were marked and handed out the door.

"To pathology," he explained for my benefit.

"The nipples," he said. I watched as, one at a time, he balanced them on his index finger and trimmed away the excess flesh with a scissor-like instrument. He folded each one into a damp cloth and set them aside.

They do this almost every day, I thought. For me it was a once-in-a-lifetime experience.

Once again the mood relaxed a moment as Pat stretched his arms and shoulders. He explained that samples from each breast were sent to pathology and that if there was no malignancy they would sew the nipples back on. If cancer was present, they would make new nipples, using pieces of skin from the very tops of the insides of the thighs and grafting them to the proper place. This would form the areola. The nipple itself was simply a trick of the trade. With a few extra stitches a sack or protrubance is made—a fake nipple.

I remembered that procedures such as these are outlined in medical textbooks just as sentence diagrams are outlined in English books, but I was no less impressed!

Sometimes I couldn't tell whose hands were whose. They worked together like a big surgical octopus with a single mind—thinking, willing, judging, perceiving, and implementing. While Pat, with the help of his assistant, was working to remove the breasts, two others were trimming skin from stomach tissue and tying off veins. They traded places as Pat stepped in to accomplish another task.

A bluesy Memphis song was playing . . . and my goodness! I was practically hanging over their shoulders!

"Tell me if I get in your way," I said as I circled the room to watch from a different perspective.

I moved to stand by the anesthesiologist and watch a small accordion in a jar. The tune it played was *beep, beep, beep*. There were two cylinders that appeared to be filled with oatmeal. Probably not.

His gaze intent on his gauges and notetaking, this doctor of sleep missed nothing. His big brown eyes—all that showed between mask and cap—were as interesting as the apparatus he was so carefully monitoring.

"This is a pulse oximeter . . . measures the saturation of oxygen in the blood . . . new in the last six or seven years . . . life saver . . . catastrophic possibilities before!" He explained his bailiwick to me in unfinished sentences, his attention never straying from the dials and gauges. I looked over his shoulder and saw the perfectly written notes on the chart.

I could only think of dumb questions like why the patient has to take off her fingernail polish prior to surgery. I've been told it's because the anesthesiologist looks at your nails to determine whether you are getting enough oxygen. He hadn't looked at her sheet-encased fingers once! Wouldn't it be funny if the new oximeter made the check-the-fingernail method obsolete and they forgot to tell Big Nurse Battle-ax?

Having made a complete circle around the room, I stopped at the foot of the table. What a dramatic view! It was like looking into a cavern. The patient's torso was wide open—held by what appeared to be an old-fashioned meat hook. I was not one bit grossed out. In fact, I recognized that a tunnel was being forged. I was enthralled at the beauty of the inside of the human body. A verse of Scripture popped into my mind:

I will praise You, for I am fearfully and wonderfully made; Marvelous are Your works. (Ps. 139:14)

Colorfully made too! There must have been twenty shades of red, from vivid coral to the palest pink, and every hue in between. The bright color of blood, I expected. What I didn't expect were reds as varied as a lipstick display. And who would have thought there'd be yellow . . . an abundance of yellow and the creamiest cream I could ever have imagined. These weren't innards; this was art! If I could capture the scene inside that cavity on canvas, it could hang in the Museum of Modern Art.

I pondered the Scripture again, and suddenly I wanted to shout it out, but the timing wasn't right, to say the least! It was quiet again but for the private language of the operating room. They seemed to understand each other, but to me it sounded like a tribal language.

"Ush shoon n tupa unna umphaz." Barely a whisper but the circulator hurried to adjust Pat's headlight once again. The air was thick with serious business. I watched amazed as hunks of stomach were tunneled through the passageway, bringing with them a blood supply vital to the success of the journey.

"Sue, look at this." I bent over Pat's shoulder to see him pull flaps of skin over each mound of tissue. Voila! It looked like breasts to me. The clock read 10:46.24.

"Nose itchin' like crazy." This time I understood the words. Pat was gesturing frantically, his gooey latex-gloved hands in the air. His surgical nurse, also with gooey latex-gloved hands, rushed to his side, and he rubbed his nose hard against her shoulder. "Ah, better!" The tension was broken for a moment, and then once again they concentrated on their work. Not a word or a motion wasted.

By now I had noticed a pattern. Total silence was in order when they cut, and minimal chatter was permitted when they stitched. Once in a while, between tasks, there was a semblance of actual conversation and an occasional joke. They continued their stitching and they braced their elbows wherever they could to get the best angle—against rib cage, thigh, shoulder—wherever.

A-ha! I thought as I remembered the many unexplainable sore spots in my body after reconstructive surgery.

The phone rang and the receiver was held to Pat's ear. "Frozen section's benign," he said to no one in particular. "Go tell her husband there's no cancer. Tell him we're almost finished and I'll be up to talk to him when I'm done. Let's have some Christmas music." The mood became festive.

Like Santa's elves they stitched—two working on the stomach area, Pat and his assistant hard at work on the breasts. Someone was whistling softly behind his mask.

They used circular needles, shaped like a big *C,* just like the ones I used in hat-making class years ago. I never got the hang of it. I couldn't imagine it in latex gloves.

The nipples were removed from their safekeeping in the damp napkins and placed in their proper position. Pat's agile fingers formed the tiny stitches . . . so perfect, so uniform. It seemed to take forever. My body was tense, as though the responsibility for the outcome was on my shoulders alone. The last stitch was finally taken, and the operating table was positioned to put the patient in a semi-sitting position. Everyone moved to the foot of the table. I was motioned along. We admired our accomplishments. Someone took a picture.

"Perfect! Good job. Nice work." Everyone was congratulating each other. I held myself back. It was probably not appropriate to cheer. I thanked everyone over and over as I pulled off my scrubs. I was supposed to take a break, call the office, and return phone calls, but I had been so captivated I forgot.

I made it to the parking garage before the impact of it all hit me. I stepped into the elevator with four other people and was about to confide what a rough morning I'd had due to the extraordinary surgery "we" just performed, when the man nearest the controls turned to me expectantly.

"Floor?" he questioned. I didn't have the slightest idea where I had parked my car or if I even had a car. My mind was blank. Finally, I recovered enough to blurt out a number and then tried to appear nonchalant as, each time the door opened, I looked desperately for my car. I went all the way to the roof and back, getting off on each floor. Finally I remembered I was parked in the basement. By the time I reached my car my legs had turned to jelly. I fumbled with the lock and managed to get myself inside where I broke out in a cold sweat.

I survived the knife, the sight of blood, the meat hook, and the rest, I thought, *and now I'm going to pass out.*

I must have sat in my car for twenty minutes before I started the motor. I was overwhelmed to think that the surgery on my own body had been almost identical to what I had just watched. The only difference was the diagnosis; mine was cancerous. I thought of the responsibility borne by the doctor and his assistants and the hospital. I remembered my surgeon, the one I'd made fun of so often. He was dead—dead of AIDS, presumably because he took on responsibility of treating patients no one else wanted anything to do with.

It never occurred to me until that day what it might be like to be accountable to a patient, to a patient's family, to the community, and to God for a human life.

The next day I went by to visit the patient. She was propped up in bed and surrounded by family. We chatted as though we were old friends.

"I had no idea I would feel this good. Dr. Maxwell was in earlier and says I'm doing great! Speaking of great, he's great . . . and this place is great," she chattered. I'd learned it wasn't unusual to hear a patient express praise for both Pat and the beautiful designer-decorated suites in the plastic surgery area of the hospital.

"How do you know him so well?" she asked. Her question gave me the opportunity to tell my favorite Pat Maxwell story that never failed to get a laugh. "All the women who know him are in love with him." I said. I explained that I'd seen many a woman flat on her back in the hospital, at death's door, pale as a ghost, breathing her last breath, the death rattle in her throat. "Suddenly through her semi-conscious daze she hears the words, 'Dr. Maxwell is coming down the hall.' She sits up, does a complete makeup job, styles her hair, sprays her best perfume, dons her best nightie, and strikes a glamorous pose!"

On the serious side, I explained that I had produced a multi-image presentation for the grand opening of The Institute for Aesthetic and Reconstructive Surgery and had been privileged to work closely with Pat; his associate, Jack Fisher; and their staff and also that we had all traveled to Washington, D.C. to meet with our congressional representatives on breast implant issues.

She glanced down at her chest. "I can't wait to see 'em. The first thing I'm going to do when these [she pointed to her bandages] come off is buy a bathing suit."

I could understand that. After all, that's exactly what I did, buy a bathing suit. I'll never forget the circumstances surrounding or following the first time I wore it.

I was self-conscious when I sunned by the pool at the magnificent Anatole Hotel in Dallas. *Should I even be wearing a bathing suit much less a two-piece suit?* I wondered. Afterward I bathed, dressed, and took the elevator down to the hotel lobby. I felt wonderful! I felt like a new person. I was a new person. I threw my shoulders back at the thought of my newly constructed body. With my clothes on, I knew I looked better than I'd looked before. I had beautiful new breasts and a flat tummy.

As I walked across the elegent oriental carpets I stopped to talk to friends. These were more than business acquaintances; these were folks we'd worked with for years. We produced their annual meetings, doing multi-image extravaganzas, video, and speech writing, and being part of the team that gave birth to concepts that would propel this Fortune 500 company through another year.

"Join us," my friends invited. As I took my seat, a very nice looking man, perhaps ten years my junior, turned to me and introduced himself. "We haven't met, but I saw you at the pool this afternoon in that pink bathing suit. You looked so pretty." I glanced at Kate, who knew my story. She winked.

There are those who might say the Lord wouldn't hear

the grateful prayer of a vain woman who has just had a strange man make a personal remark in a hotel lobby. Perhaps not, but I did utter a silent prayer of thanksgiving: *Thank You Lord, for this affirmation. You know how much I needed it. Dr. Maxwell might have remade me, but I know who did the original construction work, right down to the blueprints. Amen.*

Having new breasts is better than having a new dress or new draperies. I found myself showing them off to any female friend who appeared to be interested. One friend was out of town when I had my reconstructive surgery. The minute she got home, she dialed my number.

"How do they look? I can't wait to see. What are you doing right now? I'll be right over." I finally managed to get a word in to say that Wayne was out of town and I was starved and why didn't we meet at Dalt's restaurant for a bite to eat. "Then we can run over to your house and I can see your new body," she replied.

Fifteen minutes later when I arrived at Dalt's, she was already seated and grinning from ear to ear. Before I could scoot into my side of the booth, she was on her feet and hopping around like a Pooh bear, leading the way to the ladies' room and straight into one of the miniature stalls.

She pulled my purse from my shoulder onto her own, put her hands on her hips, and waited with anticipation as I unbuttoned my shirt and pulled it open with a flourish.

"Ta-da!" I said as I threw out my underwearless chest. "Wha'da ya think?"

"They are beautiful. Just beautiful!" she exclaimed.

"Feel them. They feel so natural," I encouraged, and she reached out, poking here and there, oohing and ahhing over my new breasts.

"They feel natural just like mine," she said. A few years before, I'd sat by her bedside after breast surgery, not because she had had a mastectomy, but because she was flat as a pancake and wanted breasts. Not bigger breasts, just breasts! It wasn't a secret; I'd seen her breasts before and after, so what happened next seemed quite natural.

"Feel mine," she said as she pulled up her shirt.

"You're right. They do feel the same," I agreed. "They really feel natural."

"We're sure fortunate, aren't we?" We adjusted our bodices and were shaking our heads at the wonder of it all as we opened the door of the stall and walked into five—count 'em—teeny boppers standing in a line, eyes wide, mouths gaping. They had obviously heard every word we had said, and we were everything their mothers had warned them about.

Show me a woman with implants and I'll show you an exhibitionist. Modest women become brazen when it comes to new breasts, and it's not at all unusual for a group of grown women to play "I'll show you mine, if you show me yours" simply because we never quite get over the wonder of it all.

I've never had a problem with my implants, and I've come to the happy conclusion that women with implants aren't dropping like flies as the media would have us believe. In the nine years since my surgery I've talked to hundreds of women who have them, and I only know of two women who have had problems. My friend Patty woke up one morning, looked in the mirror, and realized one of her saline implants had gone flat. She called her doctor, scheduled day surgery to have it replaced, and that was that. In her words, "I had a flat tire and I got it fixed." The other person with problems had a doctor who had never done the procedure. Not only wasn't he board certified, but he wasn't even a plastic surgeon!

It seems to me implants should be available for mastectomy patients and for those who simply want bigger breasts, and it should be a woman's choice. The federal government has other ideas. They've decided women need to be protected from implants, even though only a small percentage have problems. If the government would be consistent, maybe I could understand. For instance, there is an *absolute* cause and effect between alcohol and tobacco and the death rate, and yet the FDA doesn't pull liquor and cigarettes off the market; and it certainly doesn't ask users to sign releases and fill out forms so they can keep track of them, which a person has to do to get implants. I believe the patient should be educated to the risks and should be tracked, but I think the choice should be voluntary.

Continual scares by the media and the unreasonable FDA controls have caused manufacturers to pull out of the market, thus slowing research and development to a snail's pace. Insurance carriers, eager for disclaimers, are rethinking coverage, and greedy lawyers are pushing patients into litigation. Women are in limbo, second-guessing their own decisions and those of their doctors. The tragedy may be that the next generation (my own daughters included) will avoid self-examination and mammograms because reconstructive surgery is such an enigma.

My advice to a woman who is in a quandary about implants is to find an experienced, board-certified plastic surgeon, talk through the options and risks, and then make an informed decision. While you are there learn about other procedures that might be of interest. There are many women who wouldn't even entertain the thought, but my observation is that the positives of a good self-image outweigh the potential problems.

Chapter *13*

Milestones— A Vacation, a Party, and a Wedding

I t was a perfect gift from a perfect friend. "Make it through the year of chemo, behave yourself, and stay alive, and I'll take you to Grand Cayman," Joy promised. As the trip was planned and the time drew near, I wondered what kind of company I would be. I felt worn down, to say the least, and somewhat out of touch with reality. It was still as though life was happening in another dimension, just out of my reach. I could see it and hear it, but not quite be a part of it.

No sooner had we arrived at our condominium than Joy asked if I'd like to learn to snorkel. "Yea, er, sure . . . sounds fun," I answered, not wanting to disappoint her. She didn't seem to notice how unenthusiastic I was. "First thing in the morning," she said like a first-grade teacher.

The next morning I had my first and only snorkel lesson—in the swimming pool. Either I was a fast learner or Joy was a good teacher. Perhaps both. I was good! And I was ready to spend the day snorkeling—in the swimming pool! Joy had other ideas.

"See that dark area out there?" she asked, pointing out to sea. "Think you can swim that far? That's a reef, and the snorkeling there is great. Your flippers will propel you through the water pretty fast, and I'm a strong swimmer; I can save you if you start to drown."

"I barely swim," I answered, "I'll give it a try." I kept worrying that I would disappoint her; after all she had spent a lot of money on this trip, and I knew snorkeling was important to her. Off we started. I was amazed at the help the flippers gave me, and we truly did glide through the water. It didn't take long to be so caught up with the underwater panorama that I forgot my ineptness at swimming.

Nothing prepares you for some moments in life. Seeing the underwater world—a reef and the sea life it sustains—for the first time was an experience I'll never forget. The colors were spectacularly brilliant, almost neon. It seemed I was not only seeing colors and hues previously unknown to me, but new kinds of vegetation and creatures as well. It was a whole new world I hadn't even known exists.

We must've seen hundreds of types of fish. Joy wore a waterproof card attached to her wrist that helped us identify the various marine species, from octopus, to flounder, to needlefish, to barracuda, to parrot fish. We managed to *talk* underwater through the air tubes.

". . . orn ih," Joy would say as she pointed to a colorful, nubby fish and then to the corn fish on the card. Sometimes we stopped, stuck our heads out of the water, pulled off our snorkels, and had a real conversation—and I didn't sink! I couldn't believe how buoyed up I felt, almost as if a magical power was undergirding me. I didn't even have to tread water.

"I can't believe I'm doing this," I said. "I really don't swim much at all. I have no idea why I'm not sinking." Joy's eyes went to the front of my bathing suit where the left side seemed to buoy up, practically under my chin. I glanced down as my thoughts caught up with hers.

"Do you think *that's* what's holding me up?" I pointed to my bosom. "Let's find out!" With one swoop I grabbed my prosthesis out of my bodice and tossed it in Joy's direction. The next thing I knew, I was going down, as my "breast" was heading in the direction of South America.

Disregarding my mouthpiece, I gulped an enormous mouthful of saltwater, before I remembered to use my trusty flippers to propel me back to the surface. I came up sputtering and frantically glanced toward shore, only to see hotels that looked like miniature markers from a Monopoly game and sunbathers the size of gnats.

Fortunately, Joy was able to save me and my "breast," practically at the same time, but by then I was sure I couldn't possibly make it back to land.

How did I swim this far? I thought as I held on for dear life to the artificial breast with both hands, *and how will I ever get back to land?* Finally I managed to poke the prosthesis back in my bra and flail my way back. I fell face first in the sand and panted like a dog after a Frisbee game. I thought every breath would be my last, but it occurred to me that it would be far more dramatic to die snorkeling than to die of cancer.

The next day I was ready to try again. This time we went out on a diveboat; we could snorkle and then climb aboard for a rest and then snorkle again. We dove for conch, which the captain marinated and served with crackers; swam with stingrays; and were frightened out of our wits by a shark, which the captain described as the largest he'd seen inside the reef. I could picture the headlines: "Nashville woman battles killer shark and loses." Again, it seemed more heroic than dying of cancer!

The week went too fast! We walked the beach and gathered shells, talked, and gave each other facials. We fixed tuna salad one night, mashed potatoes and cooked carrots the next; the third, we visited the Grand Old House, where we ordered one of each, and charged more than we should have to our American Express cards. That night we slept on the screened porch and awakened early to the crashing sounds of the ocean.

Until my week in Grand Cayman, my whole psyche was an out-of-whack camera, and the image through the viewfinder was a blurred, distorted refraction of light and movement. Cayman was the repair shop that restored my capacity to focus. The vivid primary colors of the windsurfers against the greens of the ocean jumped at me. My sensitivities returned, and I can still remember the contrasting feelings in my body—skin burning hot from the driving sun and then tremulous shivers as I saturated myself with the chilling aloe lotion.

The tingling, slightly painful peel of a facial mask brought back other forgotten sensations—the thudding of my heart against my innards as the shark swept through the waters; the ocean pulling me down, down, down; the clinging to that stupid artificial breast and knowing I'd hang on as long as necessary because *I wanted to live*. These intense feelings became the talisman of my recovery!

There have been other trips to Cayman, with other friends, and once with our daughters. Hilarious times! But that first visit stands out as a milestone, almost as though I came back from the dead.

Another milestone was the surprise party my friends gave to celebrate my five-year survival. Our invitation said, "Please come to a listening party for new recording artists—Sunday afternoon at 3:00." Little did I know it was one of a kind, designed to throw me off the track. The rest of the guests received an invitation to a Celebrate Life! party in my honor. They were also invited to bring their art collections or handiwork for display.

Dan and Phyllis had come from Chicago to spend the weekend with us—actually to attend the party—and I apologized to them for the interruption. "We're always having to go to listening parties, but it's fine for you to go with us," I explained. "It may even be fun. You never know who will show up at these things."

As we walked through the door of the beautifully restored building on Second Avenue, cameras flashed in our direction, and I caught sight of banners proclaiming CELEBRATE LIFE! It took me a moment to realize I was looking into the faces of at least a hundred of my best friends who were cheering and smiling from ear to ear! As I turned to Wayne, the look on his face was priceless. He had known all along and had kept the secret!

A harpist played, and several young friends clad in tuxedos served hors d'oeuvres, while Wayne and I tried to take it all in. Many of my friends had been there all day hanging a gallery. The exposed brick of the old building was a perfect backdrop for Bob McConnell's works of art, Shana's black and white photography, and Leigh's oil paintings. There was poetry by Suzanne Gaither, and a large poster that proclaimed SUESATIONAL! from my friend Arch, who is a public relations executive. Mindy displayed a piece of her marbleized furniture.

From Doug and Laura Oldham there were framed pictures from another creative party we had shared years before, a Turkey Awards at which gold turkeys were given to some of the top names in music for their best-left-untold most embarrassing moments.

There was a wall hanging and matching T-shirt from Bill and Gloria, and a hand-embroidered and appliqued sweatshirt from Kay, all in the Celebrate Life motif. Joy and Peggy stood proudly beside their creation—a life-size op-art junk sculpture which looked better than some of the things I've seen in the Metropolitan Museum of Art! Joy had also made a seascape panorama, complete with sand and sea shells, that had a little plastic image of me in my pink bathing suit made from an actual photograph. Minnie's display was a bikini-torso cake just like the one she made when I was in the hospital.

We oohed and aahed and stuffed ourselves with Marty and John Coates' gourmet delights, and just when it seemed too good to be true, the crowd turned hostile! They roasted me! One by one they told their stories and poked good-natured fun at me. My brother Jon showed a video he had edited to the song "She's Got Personality." He used footage that made me want to crawl under a rug!

A group of my professional musician friends, led by Lynn Hodges, sang a song called, "She Did Her Very Breast!" which they had written, and presented me with a T-shirt with those words.

My songwriter friend, Bill Gaither, wrote a poem likening me to Tammy Faye Bakker, an overly made-up, bizarre little woman, who was once a Christian television show host. And if this weren't enough, there were gifts for me and for Wayne too—it was his birthday. The afternoon ended with some serious moments of singing and thanksgiving. Our smile muscles ached.

Recently we celebrated another significant milestone. This time, Wayne and I threw the party, and our friends and relatives came from all over the country. It wasn't officially in honor of my ten-year survival, yet as we made our plans, I couldn't help but think about it. Officially, it was the celebration of our daughter's wedding. After twelve years of being each other's best friend, it was love at first sight for Dana and Barry.

Barry's mother, Bonnie, and I tease them that we knew years ago, when they were in college, that it was a perfect match. We remind them of how we kept our mouths shut and didn't try to interfere. Through the years we watched them console each other through many failed romances, and we observed that they were obviously happier together than at any other time.

At last, "after much prayer and fasting on the part of the mothers" (Bonnie's words), Dana turned around as Barry came toward her on the ski slope, and their hearts did flip-flops. The wedding was everything we could have dreamed of. The service itself was a glorious worship experience followed by a party, a reception that none of us will ever forget. After the wedding, friends and relatives from both families changed into casual clothes and came to our house for the evening. My dear friend and right arm, Bea, helped me serve a buffet dinner, and then we all crowded into our family room to sing around the piano. From raucous hand-clapping songs to "Amazing Grace," the harmony was magnificent. Someone suggested a solo from Miles, Barry's dad who is an accomplished musician. Next we had an impromptu male quartet, then a piano solo from Matt, followed by a number by the Hines family, and on and on. My cousin's wife, Rita, played with flair any song that was mentioned, including accompanying Peggy's rowdy performance of "I'm Jest a Girl Who Cain't Say No!" from the musical, *Oklahoma*.

As the evening drew to a close, there was still one song to be sung. It would be the rousing old gospel song that had ended our family gatherings long ago. As I looked into the faces of Nancy and Jim, my cousins, I was momentarily transported back to their parents' farm in southern Ohio where we, the city cousins, visited the country cousins. I could almost see their parents—Dewey in his bib overalls and Chrissy with her mandolin in her lap—and the faces of my mother and daddy. I could almost hear all of us singing and, in memory, our harmony was perfect!

Now here we were so many years later, with our husbands and wives and children and friends. This must be a little hint of what heaven will be like, I thought to myself. Just so much joy, we can hardly contain ourselves! As if on cue, Rita struck a chord and we sang "There's going to be a meeting in the air."

Chapter *14*

A Yellow Convertible and a Pink and Black Ford

A life-threatening experience makes you look at life in an entirely new light. You become a philosopher, a theologian, a poet. You want to know where you came from, why you're here, and why you are the way you are.

What is truth? you ask. *What can I really stake my life on?* You examine the things you've been taught and try to sort truth from myth. You wonder about your roots, your history. *Who were those ancestors in the sepia-toned pictures, and what genetic characteristics were transmitted down the blood line to me? What strengths? What weaknesses? What dispositions? Predispositions?*

There is a new dichotomous perspective to your examinations. You find you are more outgoing, yet more introspective. More fearful, yet more daring. On one hand you cling more tightly to your loved ones, and on the other, you release them, knowing your hold is temporal. In many ways you are more open. You reach out to others, are more gregarious; yet at the same time you hold back, are more private. Sometimes you seem to be looking at the world from a safe distance rather than actually participating in it.

After my chemotherapy was finished, I was overwhelmed that it was over and that I was alive. I seemed to view the world in the terms of my trade, photography. I wondered if any other living person saw what I saw, felt what I felt, experienced it so deeply. My journal from that time reflects my feelings.

Today I see a paper sculpture as I look across the landscape—monochromatic grays, not a color in sight. Before I would have said, *Such a gray, gray day.* Today I say, *If it were possible to capture this, I could sell it to a king.*

The whole weekend was filled with color and motion . . . high-speed film motion! Even with the proper film there could possibly be a blur . . . horizontally across the image. Perhaps the blur would add to the magic. The sky is bluer than blue, as though you are using your polarizing filter to the max. The clouds move like shadow dancers—like visible spirits looking for a place to light. Spirits can't be photographed.

It's the magic hour—the only perfect time of the day for a photographer, when the daytime glare is gone, and there are no harsh shadows . . . just before dusk (or right after dawn if you're up!). If you shoot fast, *right now,* the pictures will be incredible in the magical lighting.

Rain . . . summer rain! With slow-speed film I could record each drop and each water-laden leaf and flower . . . drooping almost to the ground.

Construction workers . . . with ecru skin, in yellow hats . . . bright yellow like daffodils . . . their tools a creative milieu on the ground around them. Hold that shot guys!

It's a dull, dreary day they say. Dear God—it's a day! It's brittle maybe . . . winter brittle . . . but there are tinges of gold and magenta off in the distance. And there are patterns! Patterns etched in the sky and on the ground. It could be shot in color . . . subtle and pale. Perhaps black and white is better . . . to do justice to the patterns!

With a tripod I could capture the lightning. To a photographer's mind, life swirls like those thunderheads in the distance.

Not only did I feel the need to philosophize, but I wanted desperately to go home—back to Charleston, West Virginia, and retrace my steps. It probably had nothing to do with my illness; more likely my age. I've noticed that my husband and my friends have the urge to return to where they came from. Joy went back to Petoskey, Michigan, for a visit, right out of the blue. She looked up all of her mother's friends and went to the church her father pastored when she was a teenager. Wayne loves to go back to Dana, Indiana, every chance he gets. He drives through the countryside and visits his friends the Hesses, the Cheeserights, and the others.

"That's where the high school was," he says with pride, "right on that empty lot by the Methodist church." He tells me where Overpeck's store was, and where Hammerslys had their gas station. In a couple hours' time, he can take me on a tour of the whole town and remind me that all of it was his paper route once upon a time. Anyone else could give the tour in six minutes flat.

Even before the announcement came for my high school reunion, I'd been thinking about going to Charleston. Not only did I want to go to Daddy's grave, but I was feeling sentimental about people and places.

—Journal Entry—

June 1985

A trip to Charleston! Who could possibly be excited about going back to that dismal chemical valley in West Virginia? Me, that's who! It's my home! I haven't been there for years. Why am I going? To follow the compelling urge to visit my father's grave? To say thank you to the old folks (they might not be around much longer) who helped shape my life? To attend my thirty-year high school reunion?

Is it because I'm vain and want to show off? I read somewhere that the number one reason people attend their school reunions is to show that they've succeeded. I close my eyes and think about the black silk Christian Dior (designed to show just a hint of my newly created bosom) carefully folded in tissue paper in my suitcase.

"Fasten your seat belts, and bring your seat backs to an upright position for landing," the flight attendant's voice orders. "We'll be on the ground in Charleston momentarily." I press my nose to the window and see nothing.

I'm here to review the signposts of my life, and to grieve for the ones no longer here. A thousand thoughts flash through my mind. Whatever happened to Margarite and Capey? Did Capey ever build his television set? I think of Clurey and the kids I played with on Sixth Street—Lee and Francie, the Jones kids, the Liebles, and Bucky Rutledge . . . Hide and Go Seek in the lumber yard . . . helping ourselves to watermelons from boxcars on the railroad siding.

The church . . . Will I feel comfortable there? What will they say? "She's a painted woman? A painted woman can't serve the Lord!" Still, there are those I must see: Miss Anna and Miss Mattie, Jimmy, the Hugharts, Aunt Florence, Lib, the Bupps, the Gardners, the Lees. I run my hands over my bleached hair. Somehow I know it will be okay.

"Do you think the pilot can hit the runway?" my seat mate asks. "If he misses, it's a long way down." I remember that exact thing being said years ago when I flew in from college and then again when I came home with a pink bundle in my lap.

We're circling. (Perhaps he's getting up his nerve.) I remember when this airport was built. They took the tops from three mountains and filled in the valleys.

I guess the pilot has to hit the runway, no matter where it is, I think.

My rental car is in the fourth stall from the door. Driving Kanawha Boulevard to the hotel, I shun the expressway that wasn't here before. By night, things haven't changed much.

This morning, by the light of day, how different everything looks! Progress! Why couldn't they have made progress somewhere else and left my hometown alone? I look out the window and try to get my bearings. The hotel, a high-rise Marriott, seems to stand on the spot of the old Union Mission where I went as a child to hear the Fisk Jubilee Singers and see Marjoe, the boy evangelist.

I get in my rented car . . . mmmn, not dismal after all! Clusters of townhouses, and strange new towers of glass and steel, and a shopping center, smack in the middle of town!

The state capitol with its gold-leafed dome shines brightly in the sunlight.

My car heads for Sixth Street, back to my childhood home. Is this why I came back? To find my childhood? It's hard to figure out which house is mine. I have to count back from the corner. One . . . two . . . three. The old porch must have fallen down. A new façade is in its place. The hedge by the Catholic Church, where Daddy left his coffee cup every morning, on the way to the bus stop, is gone. He wedged it into the stiff branches; it was my responsibility to find it and bring it home.

The nerve of them to close Jolly's, the little grocery store where we stood in line for hours to buy bubble gum! Those were war years, and bubble gum was almost impossible to get. I giggle as I pass Sacred Heart Church, remembering Mrs. Vandertweezers and her close call with Father Cuthbert. Sixth Street Methodist Church, where we attended early on, looks just as it did. So does Bucky Rutledge's house. I remember the scarlet fever quarantine signs nailed to those pillars; signs put there by the city as a warning to all who passed. Scarlet fever! Those were dreadful words. How it frightened our mothers.

They cured that, I think, *and TB, and polio! Someday there will be a cure for cancer.*

The house on Mathews Avenue, where we lived next, will be easy to spot . . . that pretty white house with the picket fence, and the pink dogwood tree . . . big awning over the porch, with comfortable furniture, and blooming pots (I can actually picture myself sitting in the glider with Ray Harbour). Maybe I've come back to find my youth.

The description is only in my memory! I'm angry! Angry because time simply refused to stand still! My house is *pink!*—the worst shade of pink I've ever seen. And it's small. It shrank! The fence is gone. The dogwood is gone. Ray is gone.

Shall I knock on the door and see what they've done to the innards of my house? Is it pink inside too? Is the breakfast nook there? How about the bedrooms that fit up under the slant of the roof? I glance at the grass growing high between the cracks in the driveway.

That's where Wayne asked for my hand in marriage, I think and it makes me smile. We were sitting in the car with my parents, having just returned from church. *I want to marry your daughter,* . . . seems like I can almost hear Wayne's voice. Then silence! Dead silence! *Daddy, say something!* The memory makes me laugh.

Wouldn't it be funny if Daddy's gourds are still growing up over the garage? I wonder and impulsively decide to check it out. No gourds are visible, but I'm delirious that the vine is still there. It dawns on me someone might look out the window and wonder what I'm doing here, why I'm laughing.

I vow that this house where I was nurtured and loved will remain white and lovely, the fence and dogwood in place. I drive the route to my best friend's house and come back and drive my old route to Woodrow Wilson Junior High School. It's closed, boarded up like a ghost town. I drive to Stonewall Jackson High School and discover it's now a technical school.

—The Reunion—
Night One

My high school reunion! Here we all are, having come from California, South Bend, Florida, Hawaii, Chandlers Branch, and Beech Avenue. Former football captains, cheerleaders, beer drinkers, flunkies, and tuba players. I can barely remember who was who.

I'm given a name tag with a picture that couldn't possibly have been me, a skinnynecked brunette with pointy, horn-rimmed glasses. Tonight is a mixer, and it's fun to see what the ravages of time have done—or not done—to these *kids*. I'm surprised to remember that many of us were classmates from first grade to twelfth. I thought we might not know each other. It's funny how we nerdy little people turned out to be such fine adults. I'm having a wonderful time!

There are pictures on a table with a hand-lettered sign IN MEMORY OF Johnny Huff, the class clown. "Suicide," my friend tells me. My eyes skim the names and photos 'til they rest on three pictures side by side; three of my best girlfriends.

"All three died of breast cancer," someone tells me, and my thoughts go wild wondering what we all did, what we unknowingly exposed ourselves to. Was it coincidence, nothing more? It dampens my spirits.

—Morning—
Day Two

This morning I awaken early. Today I go to the cemetery. Betty, Daddy's beautiful, forever-young cousin goes with me. Her mother and daddy, Mae and Elmer, are buried nearby. We have lots to talk about, and I'm glad she's with me. I don't want to be alone. I'm so sad my parents don't rest together side by side. I think of Mother in that sandy, lonely, unshaded grave in Lantana, Florida . . . home of the *National Enquirer!* I lay my bouquet against the headstone. Is this why I'm here?

—Reunion—
Night Two

Dinner and dance. The committee has worked hard, dug up film from our senior picnic, organized the cheerleaders and majorettes for a routine, bought prizes for those with the most children, the person coming the farthest distance, etc., etc. And the person most changed . . . *me!*

There are mini-reunions around the room, bragging about children and grandchildren, and listening to the band. I dance to make up for the dancing I missed thirty years ago. God *doesn't* strike me dead. Some of my partners have had successes. Some have had none since the pass that won the football game. None have been on Donahue or Oprah. If this is why I'm here, it doesn't seem very important anymore.

Shall I go back for my fortieth reunion? We'll have to wait and see how the face-lift turns out!

—Church—
Day Three

Sunday morning I dress for church, wondering how it will be. I drive the winding road to the new location. The building is beautiful, just like a *real* church, steeple, stained glass, and all. The service is formal, but not stuffy. The music is magnificent. I see new faces, young families, children everywhere, and brightly dressed women with up-to-date hairdos! Tastefully made-up faces! I see people I remember from my youth, older but the same, and they are as happy to see me as I am to see them.

One thing is the same—exactly the same! Everyone has a Bible, and when a Scripture is mentioned, you can hear the rustle of pages turning like leaves blowing in the wind! The sound fills me with joy! I turn in my seat to look in the faces of the church people and it comes to me: *This is why I'm here!* This is truth! It was truth thirty years ago—or three hundred years ago for that matter—and it's still truth today!

I had opportunities for other reunions over the next couple of years, one with my college friends and the other with my high school friends.

When I went back to my college I kept no journal. I was there on business. I'd been asked to produce two videos for them. One was targeted to prospective students for recruitment; the second was to be used for fund-raising.

I was on campus with scriptwriters and film crews several times, once during homecoming. Beforehand, I got in touch with Liz, Ginger, and Lois and invited them to share my hotel suite with me.

To say we picked up where we left off is an understatement. It took about five minutes for the hotel rooms to look very much like our dorm rooms umpteen-dozen years before—clothes thrown everywhere and all the electrical plugs maxed out with irons, hair dryers, and curling irons. We took *beaucoup* pictures and constantly played the inevitable game of *remember when?*

"Ginger, remember when we both wanted Jack Cromer?" She remembers! "Ginger, *you* can have him!" "No, *you* take him—I insist!" We're rolling in the floor with laughter!

Liz, Ginger, Lois, and I have been in regular contact and have repeated our reunion weekend several times since.

Then there's the gang from high school years. Until our high school reunion, I hadn't seen Carlene for years. That night she, her husband Jackie, and I sat together at dinner.

"We should get the trio together," Carlene suggested. That night we made plans to call Janet, the other member of the Youth for Christ trio, and see what we could work out. Janet and I had stayed close through the years, calling each other often, and exchanging greeting cards. Once in a while I was in Dallas on business and stayed at her house.

That fall began a yearly get together of "The Trio," a bit misleading, since there are four of us. Susie took my place in the group when I went off to college; thus she qualifies as a genuine member. Each year I keep a journal of the event, and send it to the others along with pictures of our time together.

—Trio Reunion—

Year One

Once upon a weekend, four beautiful women met together in a wonderful log cabin near Dallas . . . to remember a past that binds them together for all time.

We sank into our memories just as we sank into the down sofas that first night, memories of slumber parties, egg salad sandwiches, crinolines, and Blossom Dairy, and of dreams to marry only the right man. We married the right men. We had the beautiful children we hoped for, and we *like* those beautiful children. Two of us proudly showed pictures of grandchildren. Although we had no particular ambitions in those days long ago, each of us has *become*. We are now a politician (Susie), a decorator (Janet), a songwriter and artist (Carlene), and a photographer-film producer.

We will remember this special weekend, because of a flea market, teddy bears, a huge wooden Santa, too many funnel cakes, singing in the middle of the night, and breakfast on a front porch. We'll probably never finish most of the discussions we began, never know if Fred was a passionate kisser or if Barbara ever found out the real word.

We do know that we have a rich heritage that has made us loving and compassionate women. We were blessed with Mary Cooke who patiently put up with our youthful exuberance, Walter Morrison who cheerfully drove us wherever we wanted to go, Mrs. Morrison who cooked us chicken in the middle of the night, Maynard Davis who was our conscience, kept us from singing "funeral songs," and prayed for us every morning without fail, Mrs. Staats who always wanted to go along, and Aunt Ruth whose laughter we can still hear and who made us feel always welcome.

In a poem by Stephen Vincent Benét, there is a snatch of wonderful truth that goes

> Life is not lost by dying! Life is lost
> Minute by minute, day by dragging day
> In all the thousand, small, uncaring ways,
> The smooth appeasing compromises of time . . .

If we came away with any truth, it is that each of us has discovered, or perhaps rediscovered, that we must not waste any moments. We are bound together because of a cherished past. In the future we will have some magnificent moments, and in all probability, there will be some overwhelming defeats, but we will live richer lives, assured of the love we share for each other, and we'll always remember once upon a weekend, when four beautiful women met together in a wonderful log cabin near Dallas.

Each fall since then, the four of us meet, trying to synchronize our arrivals at the Dallas airport, and drive a couple of hours north to the beautiful horse ranch with the picture-perfect guest house, where we settle in for a long weekend. Each day we make our way to First Monday in Canton, Texas, which is perhaps the world's largest flea market of antiques, teddy bears, Christmas clothing, handmade gifts, and foods. We spend three full days there and never manage to see it all.

At night we talk about old boyfriends and the cars they

drove; Eddie Starkey and the old rattletrap Chevy, Gary Monday and the yellow convertible, Ray Harbour and his pink and black Ford, and about Fred Cook, Bob Grishaber and Wesley, we-forget-his-name, and Jackie, whom Carlene did, in fact, marry. We talk about the girls we hated way back then, and Susie can still imitate Mitzy's suh-weet little whiny voice:

"It's just an ole blanket," she says. "Why, just last night my mama took an ole blanket off the bed and made this skirt. It's just an ole blanket." We laugh till we cry and then discuss whether Mitzy and Nicky could possibly still be happy together after all these years. Someone points out that he'd probably have been happier with me.

I didn't ever *want* Nicky; I just didn't want Mitzy to have him! "Sure! Sure!" they say.

We eventually turn out the light and go to bed, but not necessarily to sleep. That's when the candy bar fights begin. Before I had cancer, the four of us barely kept track of each other; now here we are acting like junior high school girls for whole weekends at a time. As our visits became more raucous, so did my journal entries!

> A rustic cabin . . . all night blabbin'
> Fallen logs . . . morning fogs
> Lots of eats . . . flowered sheets
> Rocking chairs . . . teddy bears
> Just some things that come to mind
> and we hate to leave behind!
> Talk and talk . . . yackety yacket
> Quilted shirts and quilted jackets
> Hats with dolls . . . and Siebert calls
> Chad . . . MAD!
> Cake . . . lake
> Thoughts from here and thoughts from there
> In thirty years . . . will we care?
> Bluegrass pickin' . . . cluckin' chicken
> Plastic cup . . . pull the string
> What, oh what, will next year bring?
> Happy homes and smiling faces?

Cats and pillows made with laces
Times that cannot be repeated
Thoughts that come out uncompleted.
Trio songs that make us glad
Candy man and corndog lad
Were we flirts? . . . Christmas shirts
Candy bars that fall like hail
Pelting us from o'er the rail
Loading cars with stuff and stuff
Do we know what is enough?
Ah! Such friends we all became
Remember this . . . Love is the same!

I love our secret language and knowing that we're the only four people in the whole world who understand it. I love the fact that these friends love me unconditionally and that we'll always be there for each other. Little did we know when we were together last November that Janet's husband Jim was already consumed with cancer and would be dead within seven weeks. As he did every year, he snapped our picture before we left for the airport. He looked pale and complained of a pain in his side. Later, as we scattered his ashes around the lake where he and I fished (when I was bored with shopping), I couldn't help but wonder why it had to happen. *This is Dallas*, I thought, *a city known for its medical centers. Will there ever be a cure for this disease?* This question hung over my head like a cloud as I boarded the plane for Nashville.

Chapter 15

A Quest
for the
Nobel Prize

Aunt Edna, my alter ego, often jokes about the medical profession. "My doctor complained because my check came back. I told him, 'So what? So did my arthritis!'"

Aunt Edna aside, it's no secret how we feel about doctors. Most of us have a love-hate relationship with them. We love them because we believe they know the secrets that will make us whole. On the other hand, we are mad because it's a nuisance to have to go to them, it's expensive, and let's face it, we're insecure because *they know more than we do!* It's a mystery to me that we can feel so secure in almost every area of our lives and yet feel so insecure with doctors.

For me it's like going to McDonald's. I stand there in line saying my order over and over in my head, so I won't embarrass myself when I get to the front of the line—Big Mac, small fries, a cup of water, and chocolate chip cookies. Likewise, I sit there half-naked in the examination room saying my symptoms over and over in my head like a third grader who is scared of her teacher!

I'm sure people in the medical profession have their insecurities too; it's just that most of the time they don't let them show. Some time ago I told my dentist how much I enjoyed my visits to his office and how I looked forward to talking to him. I thought the poor man was going to cry. "No one has ever said that to me before. Usually, my patients say, 'You're the last person I wanted to see today!' " He explained that after a while you want to quit. You just can't take it anymore. His words were prophetic.

One day I called his office and was told the number was no longer in service. Later I saw him in a store dressed in shabby clothes and with long unkempt hair. "I'm a dropout from society," he told me. "I'm working in the mountains of Tennessee in a program that provides free dental care for poor children. They really like me!" He told me he had never been happier.

I'll never forget Doctor Joe Selman, who brought me into the world and took care of our family until he died. He was a giant of a man with a gentle soul. We could *drop in* for a visit in his downtown office, or he would come to the house. Dr. Joe was right up there close to God when it came to respect. "He probably has more patients than anyone in town, but he never shortchanges you," mother would say. And as though she were announcing some specialty for which he had trained, she would add, "He practices common sense medicine."

The last time I saw Dr. Joe was on a visit back to Charleston when Dana was two and was suffering from an earache.

"Honey, I can prescribe something for those ears, but from what you tell me she's been living on antibiotics for the last two years. Maybe it would be best to let her little immune system begin working on its own. Let's just watch her closely and keep her fever down. Besides, I hate to stick needles in these sweet little bottoms," he said as he patted hers. I took his advice and Dana never had another earache.

Sometime between my childhood and that of my children, the family doctors, who knew us, loved us, and communicated with us, disappeared; or at best, they became few and far between. To me, the words *know* and *communicate* are like the song "Love and Marriage," they "go together like a horse and carriage."

I know a lot of doctors socially, and others I know through business connections; but it's hard these days to find one who wants to *know* me when I'm his patient. I don't want to go to his kid's bar mitzvah or have lunch with him; I just want him to know me as a person instead of a malady—a bone, a heart, or a tumor. "Hey, nurse, pull the file on that cancer with the blonde hair!"

After so many years of listening to women talk about their problems with doctors, it occurred to me that I might work towards solving the dilemma not only for myself, but for all humankind. By doing so, I might be eligible for the coveted Nobel Peace Prize. My first thought was what I would wear to accept my award. Next, I took out a piece of paper and made two columns. In the first I wrote, What Medical People Can Do, and in the second, What Patients Can Do. So far, so good! Next I gathered my data.

I began close to home with my sister-in-law, Becky, who is an radiologic technologist. She not only keeps me supplied with articles on diagnostic techniques and other interesting things about the cancer industry, but I can count on her to help me think things through. I talk to her almost every day. Sometimes I have an excuse, to get a recipe or to find out what she does to make her pansies bloom so well. Most of the time I call simply because I need a *Becky fix!* She is levelheaded and calm—two things I'm not—and I've learned to depend on her wise and thoughtful judgment.

"I'm going to ask you a question; tell me the first thing that pops into your head," I said when Becky answered the phone. I took the silence to mean she was waiting eagerly for the question. "What's the one thing a patient could do to make your job easier?" I didn't think my question funny, yet I could barely hear Becky's answer through her laughter.

"Take a bath!" she giggled. "Sometimes I have a patient who smells so bad I'm tempted to hold my nose with one hand and X-ray him with the other."

"So whataya do?" I asked.

"You do the same thing you do when you change dirty diapers; you breathe through your mouth!" We both had a good laugh, and after I hung up I wrote a poem and faxed it to Becky's office.

This lim'rick is straight from your docs;
Sometimes when you take off your sox,
The smell is so awful
It's almost unlawful.
You'd think they were treating an ox.

The doctors present this petition;
"Don't come in a dirty condition.
Wash the parts of your bod,
Or honest to God,
We'll not want to be your physician."

An unclean patient coerces
A doctor to tantrums and curses.
He'll sure go berserk
And act like a jerk
And perhaps take it out on his nurses.

Don't spray yourself down with perfume
'Cause *you* like it, please don't assume!
One person's smell
Is another one's hell,
He might dread coming into the room.

When you're in that small room and it's close-ed
And your parts are all out there expose-ed,
If the odor is rotten,
To the morgue you'll be gotten
'Cause your body has smelled decompose-ed.

We've all had mothers, I conject,
Giving unwanted advice. Is that correct?
From now until doomsday,
The one thing they all say
Is "change underwear," you might be in a wreck!

Mothers have been saying that last line almost as long as
they've been telling us not to kiss the cat, lest we get a terrible
disease. I personally have never heard of a person in a terrible
wreck, being pried free by the jaws of life, loaded on the
stretcher, bloodsoaked beyond recognition, and of hearing an
ambulance attendant say, "Look at this poor girl's underwear.
I don't believe she's changed it for a couple of days." I'm not

saying it never happened, but if so, I haven't heard about it. It could be it's the main topic of conversation at the National Ambulance Drivers' Convention.

After striking out with Becky, it occurred to me that if I interviewed a thousand physicians and asked them what the *patient* could do to bring about a better doctor-patient relationship, I would get a thousand different answers, everything from "Stop hanging my diplomas and pictures upside down!" to "Pity me! How would you like to go through life hearing your mother brag about 'my son the doctor' when what you really wanted to be was a country singer?"

If you asked a thousand patients what the *doctor* could do to improve the relationship, you would get a thousand answers, the most repeated one being, "He could read *Good Housekeeping!* After all, that's where I got my symptoms! Good doctors will run each other down getting to the newsstand to find out the latest maladies and their cures, so they'll know what they are talking about!"

Ten years ago, after my mastectomy, when I was frantically making the rounds and the phone calls to gather information, I called a shirttail relative of Mother's in Colorado. (We aren't sure about the shirttail or if there really is a connection.)

My phone call to Dr. Marvin Burnett was one of the most significant things I did. Dr. Burnett, one of six physicians at Hematology and Oncology Associates in Denver, had the unique ability to take my jumbled thoughts and help me make sense of them. I spoke to Marvin several times over the next few weeks, and while he didn't give me any earth-shattering new information, I always put down the phone with a better understanding of the strange new things that were going on in my life. Not only that, but I found him to be a fascinating conversationalist! Through the years we've been in touch a few times; once on a business trip to Denver, I had dinner with him, his wife Alison, and his mother-in-law Ruby. It was a lively and fun evening.

Not long ago, I called Marvin again, and as always

seemed to happen, the conversation turned into a good natured sparring match on the subject of doctor-patient communication.

"Marvin, let's solve it once and for all. Let's write down what medical professionals should expect from patients and vice versa, box it, and sell it on the street corner." I didn't tell him about my dream of the "Nobel!" (I didn't want to share the glory unless I had to.)

"Sue, I've told you before, and I'm tellin' you again, there's no formula . . . there are no lists." I could hear the how-many-times-do-I-have-to-tell-you implications coming through the phone line. Then he said, "Get on a plane and come out here; follow me around a couple of days. Meet the people I work with, talk with my patients, and then you'll know." We spoke again several days later, and once again Marvin urged me to come to Denver.

I had no intentions of going to Denver. I certainly enjoyed a good chat with Marvin now and then, but if I was going to use the free plane ticket in my desk drawer, it would be to talk to a person on my *hot shot* list, someone I'd seen on television or read about in the news. However, one of Marvin's comments kept replaying in my mind, and the more times I heard it, the more it made sense. "You know, Sue, about 10 percent of docs are the biggies, the media types, the ones you read about or see on television. Maybe about 5 or 10 percent are the bad guys, the ones who are doing what they do for the wrong reasons. And the rest of us, you know what we are? We're just journeymen. We work hard. We aren't after recognition. We are simply busy caring for people. Sue, you need to know what the journeymen are doing. Come on out here." I thought about Marvin's invitation often over the next few days and finally had my secretary book the flight.

This is probably a wild goose chase, I thought as I drove from the Denver airport. *Even if it is, I'll enjoy all this beauty. Where else can I see the flowering trees of spring against a backdrop of snow-capped mountain peaks?*

Even if this is a wild goose chase, at least I'm getting some busi-

ness in, I thought as I pulled into Colorado Springs to have lunch with one of my favorite clients, Dorothy Gore, vice president of Christian Booksellers Association.

At least I'm getting to spend an afternoon with a good friend I haven't seen in a while, I thought that afternoon as I walked through the shops at the famous Broadmoor Hotel with Beth Loux, whom I knew from Chicago days and who now lives in Colorado Springs.

Probably a wild goose chase, but at least it's been good to spend the evening with Ruby, admiring her beautiful oil paintings, and reminiscing together about Mother, I thought as I got ready for bed at Ruby's house.

The next morning at the crack of dawn, Marvin, coffee cup in hand, picked me up in his Jeep. He called it his Colorado Cadillac. We chatted as he dodged traffic on our twenty-minute trip to downtown Denver. "You have free rein to talk to people—office staff, nursing staff, patients. Ask questions, observe, absorb. That's what you're here for—to absorb."

He glanced at me from under the Rockies baseball cap he wore to keep his hair from blowing in the breeze from the sunroof. "When this day is over, you'll at least know the answer to one of your questions: *What should a person expect from his doctor?* I want you report to me at the end of the day and tell me what you learned." *Gee, I didn't know there would be a quiz,* I thought as we pulled into the parking garage. We made our way along the corridors to his office. I plugged in my laptop computer, and he filled our coffee cups.

"I get a card and a letter every year from a patient who was diagnosed with granulocytic leukemia when her son was born. I guess he's sixteen years old now." Marvin is shuffling through his desk. "I treated her at that time. She's been in remission all these years—chromosome cure. The disease doesn't even show up in the chromosomes." I assume Marvin's desk shuffling means he's looking for the letter to prove his case. Finally, he gives up, leans back in his chair, and smiles a satisfied smile. "That's the hole in one! That's why you come back the next day! And oh, by the way, don't forget, I want to know what answers you've found to your questions at the end of the day." With that he headed down the hall to see his first patient. *Yeah and I want naturally blonde hair too!* I said to myself.

I moseyed down the hall to the front office where a hand-lettered sign caught my attention. I stopped to read.

> Cancer is so limited . . .
> It can't cripple love,
> It can't shatter hope,
> It can't corrode faith,
> It can't eat away peace,
> It can't destroy confidence,
> It can't kill friendship,
> It can't shut out memories,
> It can't silence courage,
> It can't invade the soul,
> It can't reduce eternal life,
> It can't quench the Spirit.
> It can't lessen the power of the resurrection.

The words reminded me of something Marvin had said on the way to the office. "The person with cancer isn't a different person from before he had cancer. He is the very same person. The body is just the monument to the person. I can treat the disease, but I can't touch the *you* of you."

The nurses in the lab were busy preparing for patients, but they invited me into the cramped space. "You can come in, but your coffee cup can't. Those are government rules, not ours." We introduced ourselves.

"We were just talking about the support group that was started last week," said Joyce, a classy-looking woman with fashionably cut hair, maroon glasses, and a big smile. "It's something we've really needed."

"Oh yes," I agreed wholeheartedly. "I'm a believer in support groups. I've seen them work for hundreds of patients."

"Not them! Us!" Joyce laughed as she fooled with the gauges on a machine. Then she turned to look at me; and even though she was smiling, I could see the pain in her eyes.

"We do have support groups for patients, but we've just begun a support group for *us,* to help us deal with *our* grief. We get so attached to our patients that when we lose one—and we do lose them—we need to talk about it. We need a chance to cry. Matter of fact, the other night at the meeting, there wasn't a dry eye in the place." This was new to me. I thought medical people were supposed to hold their patients at arm's length and not become emotionally involved.

Marvin's philosophy came in bits and pieces. Each time after he saw a patient, he found me and offered another observation. "Ya know, Sue, after the diagnosis, the first thing a doctor should do is treat a person for shock. Remember what you learned when you were a Girl Scout? Treat the person for shock. We rarely begin medication on the first visit. We talk to them, listen to them, assure them. We treat 'em for shock." With that, Marvin hustled down the hall to another patient.

"Another thing, you don't try to make a patient a medical student." It was as though he hadn't left the room. Marvin had the knack of picking up right where he left off, almost in the middle of a sentence. "You give her the truth, but you don't ram it all down her throat at once. It's like telling your children about sex. You tell them as they ask. That's what you do with a patient—you answer her questions today, and then you answer her questions tomorrow, and the next and the next. Yeah, that's a lot of phone calls, a lot of time on our part," he said as though he read my mind, ". . . but that's what we're here for." Again he disappeared into an examination room.

The next time Marvin appeared it was to motion me to follow him. "Come on and go with me." I wasn't sure I was ready to meet a patient, but I didn't have time to think about it. Suddenly I was being introduced to Leigh, a breast cancer patient not much older than Mindy, and her mother, who was visiting from the East.

"Leigh has had a bone marrow transplant. That's why she's wearing a mask . . . has to guard against infection." I knew that in younger women with breast cancer, the procedure was to take out bone marrow, treat it intensively to eradicate all tumors, and then re-fuse it.

As Marvin checked his patient, much as I'd been examined by Doctor Solomon ten years before, my eyes were glued to the mother. Her body language and the pain in her beautiful face told the story well. If she could not take the place of her desperately sick daughter, then she would *feel* every horrible moment with her. Even as the doctor prodded the inside of Leigh's mouth with his tongue depressor, the woman's mouth worked the same contortions as that of her child.

When Marvin finished his examination, he sat down, and he and Leigh had a typical doctor-patient dialogue. "How have you been feeling?, . . ." "Have you been unusually tired?, . . ." "How's your appetite? . . ." "*No, it's probably not a good idea to go to a rock concert this weekend because of the chance of infection. Your white count is just too low.*"

Marvin stood and laid his hand gently on Leigh's arm. "I'll be back in a minute. The results of the blood work should be ready. I'll check . . . be right back." He gave her arm a squeeze. "I really think the concert is out, regardless. Sorry 'bout that." When the door closed behind him, Leigh turned her tired eyes to her mother. "Did you see that Mom? Did you see him put his hand on my arm? Did you see him touch me?" The mother had noticed. She had felt it too.

The news Marvin brought back wasn't good. He rattled off numbers that both women understood. "Why hasn't it come up yet? I've talked to two other patients who had bone marrow transplants, and the blood count came right back." Marvin sat down and thought a moment. "Well, how many times have you seen a pregnant woman and she tells you she's overdue, and everybody keeps saying *why hasn't it come? I don't understand*. Well, it's just not ready. It will come, though, and that's what I think about your blood count—it'll come when it gets ready. Just takes longer for some people. We have more tricks in the bag . . . we'll do a booster if we have to. That will stimulate the bone marrow to produce white cells. For now, Leigh, let's just take it a day at a time."

"You talk a little bit, you listen a little bit," Marvin tells me in the hallway. "Matter of fact, if you let a patient talk long enough, she'll tell you what is wrong."

"In that case, Marvin, I could be a doctor!"

I was surprised at how the time had flown. Before leaving for a hospice meeting, Marvin arranged for me to have lunch with Sharon, the office manager, and Ginny who is in charge of the nursing staff. As we waited for the elevator, we couldn't help but overhear the uncontrollable sobs of a woman using a pay phone. Her face was pressed tightly against the wall so as not to draw attention to herself. "We've got to do something about that. People need privacy at a time like that." I could see Ginny making a mental note to find a place for patients to make phone calls in private.

As we sat down to eat, I commented on the fact that between the two of them, Ginny and Sharon seemed to be aware of everything that went on. "Some people would have missed the lady in the hallway. After all, it must happen every day in medical offices all over the country." "Our antennae are always up," Sharon responded. "That's our number one job—to make it easier for the patient."

During lunch I learned that making it easier for the patient meant everything from coming in early in the morning to help someone get to work on time (even on a Saturday morning when patients normally aren't scheduled) to calling a cab for someone too sick to drive. "We have a tab with the cab company. If a patient calls and says he can't come in, that he's too weak to drive, we say, 'You need to be here—a cab is on the way.'"

"We also have a tab at a nearby restaurant. If a patient has to wait for tests or for reports to come back or because we just can't get to them, we buy their lunch. No one says, 'Should we arrange for that couple to have lunch? They've been here a long time.' It's just understood. It's taken care of."

After lunch I poked my head into the business office, which was much as I would have predicted: workers with computer screens full of numbers. This was something I understood. We had produced medical films explaining reimbursement procedures. I could even guess that one or two employees were doing nothing but filing Medicare claims and trying to keep up with its constantly changing guidelines.

Around the corner in a small cubbyhole, I noticed a young woman working alone. Taped along the edges of her computer screen were baby photos. I stood admiring the pictures for a few minutes, not knowing if I should interrupt. "That's my baby," the young woman offered as she turned from her screen. "Two months old! I'm Karen. I'm the study coordinator. I'm doing research." With a little prompting, I was able to find out the answer to a question that had plagued me for years: *How do doctors keep up with information?*

"We're connected into everything we need: pharmaceutical studies, the National Cancer Institute, universities, anything and everything in cancer research. I'm continually moving around in the computer world. The doctor who has a patient with a particular tumor tells me, 'Get in there and get the new studies.' I work with the patients too. I tell them about new studies, and if they qualify, I give them an opportunity to participate. There might be a new protocol that is approved by the FDA but is still on trial. I keep track of the participants and feed that information into the computer too." I thanked Karen for her time and walked out into the hallway.

Lucy and I enjoyed a good-natured banter after I discovered it was her responsibility to keep up with OSHA regulations. Because we had produced a film about it, I knew that the Occupational Health and Safety Administration regulations are the laws the government lays down for almost every industry known to man. OSHA covers everything from how to handle blood properly, to what to do in case of a chemical spill, to something as simple as how to put on and take off your latex gloves. "I think you are a subversive, Lucy," I teased. "You keep checking that big thick book that says OSHA on the cover. I think you work for *them,* that OSHA whatever it is, not the clinic." "It's not funny—it's true!" she said, and explained that her sole job is to understand, interpret, and oversee implementation of these regulations.

All day I had been hearing about Libby Tracey. "Wait till you meet *her*," they told me. "I don't know if you're ready for *her*, she's a real character!" At lunch Ginny told me about Libby's first week on the job. It seems that Libby knew it was mandatory for a nurse who works in an oncology/hematology clinic to have a blood test. Even though she was a nurse, Libby could barely stand to draw a patient's blood, much less have her own taken. "I'm warning you," Libby told them, "I won't survive!"

The next day Ginny heard her name called over the loud-speaker ordering her to the lab, STAT!, which means quick. There she saw Libby stretched out on the floor looking unconscious or worse! After a few seconds everyone burst into laughter, including the patients, who were in on the joke. From everything I was told, Libby kept the place hoppin'!

"Where is this person you've been telling me about?" I asked as I picked up the phone to call my office. "The day is almost over, the patients have gone home, and I've yet to meet this Libby person." As I was finishing my conversation with my secretary, suddenly out of nowhere appeared a tiny blonde dynamo of a person, who threw herself at me full force, hugged me like a linebacker, and plunked a kiss that hit halfway on my forehead and halfway in my eye. When I hung up the phone one second later, she was nowhere to be found. Before I could get up from my chair, she was back, this time wearing a coolie hat and dragging along Malliah, a nurse I'd met earlier. "Let's sing for Sue." Malliah is a musician who performs and records with her gospel singing family, but the only similarity between Libby's performance and show biz, as we know it, was the fact that she did look like a shorter Carol Channing.

Libby had been in class all day, her last class to complete a doctoral program in nursing, and there was great speculation as to whether her associates would be required to call her *Doctor Nurse*. When I asked about her role at H.O.A. she answered, "I'm the cheerleader." It wasn't hard to imagine she was a key ingredient there; the person who bolsters not only the staff, but the patients as well.

"Gotta run to the hospital," she said, giving me another bear hug. "I'll be there late, but I'll be joining you at Marvin's and Alison's for dinner." She was gone.

The office was quiet, and Marvin motioned for me to sit down. "So, how 'bout it Sue? Are you glad you came? Did you get your answers?" He sat with his elbows on his desk and his index fingers pointed like a church steeple at his chin.

"Yeah, Marvin. I had my answers by noon. It's so simple. What I want from you and your staff is exactly what I saw here today. I want someone to be happy my family member or friend has been free of leukemia for sixteen years, to call it a hole in one, and I want someone to be willing to go out of her way for me, maybe come in early so I can get to work on time. I want someone to notice that I need a quiet place for a phone call; maybe pay for my cab or lunch. And I'd love a cheerleader, a Libby to make me laugh in the midst of my pain. And a touch! I wouldn't mind a touch, a hand on my arm now and then. And Marvin, do you know what the most comforting thought in the world would be?" He shook his head. "To know that someone would shed a few tears if they lost me."

"It's really simple, isn't it, Sue? What we want from each other is what we want from everyone: respect . . . and kindness . . . and above all, caring. If we all had those, there wouldn't be a problem. Right?" Marvin rolled back his chair and rose to his feet. "Right!" He'd answered his own question. "Let's go home!"

Chapter 16

Dandruff, Cobwebs, and Lizard Spit

Not long after Wayne and I moved to Nashville, we were invited to a party. Afterward someone asked, "How did you like mingling with country music stars?" Fortunately my response wasn't, "What country music stars?" The truth of the matter is, I had no idea we had been in the presence of stars! The next day I decided that if I was going to live in a town affectionately known as *guitar city,* I would learn about the industry that brought it fame. I began by asking questions, reading brochures, and visiting the country music museum. I even got on a tour bus and found out where the studios are and where the stars live.

Since that time, I've had the privilege of producing multi-image shows and videos for various music and music-related companies; we've also entertained a few *stars* in our home. Now I have such appreciation for country music that all of the buttons on my car radio are programmed to country stations; and when I travel, the first thing I do when I get into my rental car is find the "twang!" Even when I was in South America for a video shoot, I listened to the "sounds of Nashville."

Where would country music be if it couldn't ask the question, Why? Why *did* he leave me? Why *doesn't* he leave me? Why'd she "do me wrong"? Why doesn't anything go right for me? And even, "Why me, Lord?" I wish I'd known about country music when I broke up with Ray and Jack. It certainly would have eased the pain!

Country music is where the rubber meets the road. It seems that just when life is going along at a pretty good clip, it happens—a severed relationship, a loved one with a drug problem, a business down the tubes, an illness, or even a death. The rain hits the crepe paper! Then come the questions: *Why my loved one? Why my business? Why didn't someone do something? Why me? Why now?*

I hear a lot of *whys* related to cancer, and I'd hoped to have all the answers before I got to the last chapter of this book. I had planned to get a couple of theological degrees and a Ph.D. or two in science. Perhaps I would become a medical doctor and get a graduate degree from fortune-telling school as well. I would spend a year in a monastery contemplating what I'd learned, and by then I would surely have the answers! It didn't work out. First of all, there simply wasn't time for the educational process; and as for the monastery, it doesn't allow Pizza Hut deliveries, time out to go to the beauty shop, or idle talk, which rules out the gossip I'm quite fond of!

One question I hear over and over in regard to cancer is, *Why can't they find a cure for this horrible disease?* For one brief moment on a flight from Nashville to Chicago, I thought I would learn the answer to that question. That night I sat next to a distinguished-looking man, who spread papers and journals out all over his lap and the seat between us.

"You look busy! Sooo, what do you do? What's all this stuff?" I asked in my most cheerful voice.

He gave me a "drop dead" look over the top of his half-framed glasses. In his most *don't bother me, lady, I have work to do voice,* he said, "I'm a scientist, and I'm making a speech in Chicago."

I can take a hint! I got *my* stuff out of *my* briefcase and spread it out all over the place. So much for conversation en route to Chicago!

He shuffled papers for a couple of minutes, probably rethinking the situation, then said, "What do *you* do?" For the next hour we talked; and when we landed, he told me he traveled every week and had never before exchanged so much as a word with a fellow passenger. He said he couldn't believe how the time had flown. Of course!

Somewhere over Indiana, I asked him to tell me, from a scientist's point of view, where we stand in cancer research and when a cure will be found. "Don't use your scientist language," I said. "Tell me in words I can understand."

He leaned back, took a sip of his Bloody Mary, and thought a while. I could see him scrambling for an explanation my blonde head could understand. "Nowhere! We're nowhere," he said.

"It's like outer space, like going to another planet. It's not the getting there that's the problem. It's the fact that when you finally get there, you not only don't have maps, but also you don't have roads. Even worse, the engineers are just beginning to survey and think things through. They're still trying to come up with first-draft blueprints." He shut his eyes a moment. "Fact is, maybe we haven't yet arrived on the moon, much less begun to figure out where roads go and why."

Unlike my seatmate on the plane, another scientist, Dr. Martin J. Murphy, Jr., president and CEO of Hipple Cancer Research Center in Dayton, Ohio, sees the proverbial cup half full rather than half empty. Given the chance, he'll talk your leg off on the subject. Erma Bombeck, who once followed Dr. Murphy at the dais, called him "a hard act to follow." He's animated, funny, and able to communicate his own compelling sense of urgency about cancer research. His perspective is not just that of a scientist, but that of a cancer patient as well.

"We're peeling away the onion," Dr. Murphy says with excitement, "layer after layer after layer." He tells me they are doing things, at least in the lab, that would have been considered science fiction four or five years ago.

I became acquainted with Dr. Murphy through his executive assistant, Bonnie Shafer, Dana's mother-in-law. At Bonnie's invitation, I visited Hipple and met some of the folks who are on the cutting edge of cancer research. Each staff member stopped to welcome me and explain his or her niche in systematic scientific investigation. Everyone seemed every bit as thrilled about his or her place in the chain of progression as an astronaut would be about walking on the moon.

Dr. Murphy is optimistic about cures for cancer, and he is careful to speak in the plural. "Cancer is many diseases," he explains, ". . . so we're talking about *cures,* not *a cure.*"

It took a long time for that concept to sink in; to understand that it isn't one singular disease, like polio or TB, and that we will never find a vaccine that will wipe out all cancer once and for all. Cancer is like the weeds in my rock gardens.

The year we moved to Nashville, Wayne built two rock gardens for me. He dragged rocks from all over the property, stacked them neatly on a natural ledge in the backyard, and brought load after load of soil up the stone steps in a wheelbarrow. It was truly a labor of love. In the spring and summer I can roll over in bed, look out the window, and admire the yellow daylilies, daisies, and those little purple flowers whose name I don't know. I like to sit on the back step with a glass of iced tea and take in the bed of begonias, impatiens, and a colorful variety of perennials and wildflowers. Every spring after the tulips have finished their show, I pull on my gardening gloves, pick up my trowel, and begin weeding.

The problem I have year after year is that I still don't always know which are the wildflowers, which are the perennials, and which are the weeds. The annuals I have down pat! They are the ones I picked up at farmers' market yesterday. If I wait too long to begin my yard work, the weeds, always greedy for nature's nutrients, will have become so thick and obnoxious that they will have taken over and the *keepers* will be puny. They may not even survive. Like the weeds, cancer's nature is to multiply, take over the garden, and choke out the flowers—the healthy cells.

Cancer is like my weeds, too, in that there are so many varieties. According to Dr. Murphy, there are more than one hundred pathologically documentable kinds of cancer; and I've read that breast cancer in young women is actually a different disease from the one that attacks older women. Even each person's cancer is different from the next and can differ in its resistance to drugs; for instance, whether or not a tumor has estrogen receptors makes a difference in its rate of growth.

"Should we find that evasive cure (the weed poison)," Dr. Murphy tells me, "it may be so toxic it will do more damage than good, seriously inhibiting the patient's ability to replenish the life-sustaining blood cells." Therefore, simultaneous with the *magic potion*, they are searching for effective *delivery boys* to take it to the site of the tumor or carry it through the bloodstream to be absorbed by the cancer cells themselves.

One of the ways this is being done is by engineering cells that can deliver the toxic substances specifically to the site of a tumor. Perhaps this is what my scientist friend on the plane meant when he referred to building roads on the moon. This is good news to those of us who have suffered the side effects of chemotherapy and the barbaric way it is implemented—like buckshot—get it out there and hope it hits something.

In the future it won't be necessary to poison the whole garden to get the weeds. We won't have to give the weeds a head start before we act, and they can be pinpointed and blasted, leaving the flowers strong to bloom and reproduce.

Until my visit to Hipple Cancer Research Center, my knowledge of science, from a class at Stonewall Jackson High School, and a because-you-have-to college lab, gave me an inaccurate mental picture of what really goes on in cancer research. I pictured a bunch of white-coated men and women mixing up an assortment of stuff in test tubes and then calling in a bunch of volunteers to try the different potions to see which ones work.

I even wondered if scientists only thought in terms of chemicals. I wondered if they ever looked for cures in common things. What if they mixed dandruff with cobwebs and the spit of a lizard? Imagine my surprise to learn that they *do* find answers in common things. For instance, by studying how chickens lay eggs, scientists are learning about a condition that results in destruction of the bone and causes elevated levels of calcium in the blood. In knowing that, they have found a way to improve the patient's life and open a window for chemotherapy to treat the cancer itself.

As far as I know, there are no known cancer cures in lizard spit, but I met Dr. Nikolaos Zilakos at Hipple, who is, in fact, experimenting with the newt, a close relative of the lizard, and is making some revolutionary discoveries. Years ago in that high school science class (or was it college?), we girls watched as the boys eagerly pulled the tails from newts. It took only a few weeks for the little guy to grow a new tail, just as science predicted!

The only method of controlling cancer today is to kill malignant cells by surgery, chemotherapy, or radiation. But by studying the regenerative tissue of that tricky little critter, the newt, Dr. Zilakos is learning revolutionary applications that hold promise and hope for tomorrow's cancer patients.

Sometimes Dr. Murphy goes on a rampage of scientific gobbledygook, and I have no idea what he's talking about. That was the case when he told me about genetic coding. I had to remind him to speak as though I were a sixth grader.

Gobbledygook aside, he's good with analogies. He compares the genetic coding of the human body to an orchestra. "If the composer, the maestro, and the musicians knew nothing about music and couldn't read it, couldn't even hear it in their heads, and couldn't play it, there would be cacophony!" Dr. Murphy wonders if the word cacophony is too much for a sixth grader and defines the word, ". . . a meaningless mixture of crashing sounds."

"But," he continues, "once you understand the code, you can learn it and work with it. Then everything changes. It's then that music can be composed, played, engineered, and understood!"

Pausing again to take note of my juvenile level of understanding, he continues: "Just as with music, there's a system to genetic coding. If there is no understanding of it, there is chaos. On the other hand, when we understand it, we can play it, engineer it!" That excites my sixth-grade understanding! "Soon the *behavior* of cells, that makes them cancerous in the first place, can be isolated, identified, and engineered—*played*, if you will." Aha! I understand! The weeds can be destroyed while they are still dormant in the ground!

Perhaps someday there will be a major breakthrough against this dreaded disease. Meanwhile, there probably isn't a cancer patient alive who hasn't had a good case of the *Why Me's?*—if not aloud in broad daylight, then surely during those long, dark hours of the night when he can't bring himself to elbow the loved one sleeping beside him or is too paralyzed to pick up the phone and cry out for help. I certainly have asked the *why me* question, not only in regard to my own illness, but to those of my parents as well.

Why did *my* parents have to die rather than our alcoholic neighbors who fought like alley cats. It wasn't that we were nosy—you would have had to be deaf to miss their Saturday night battles! Our houses were close, and in the summer when the windows were open, we could hear every word *and* every smack of Tressy's knife when it hit the stairsteps as she crawled upward. "Charles, [smack] you [smack] ole [smack] . . . [smack] I'm gonna [smack] kill you. I'm comin' up [smack] to kill you [smack] right now" [double smack].

"She'll never kill him. They'll outlive us," Mother would say. "They're probably pickled, those two!" Mother was right; Tressy and Charles outlived both my parents by many years. *Why my parents? Why not those miserable neighbors?*

Peggy, seven years after Bob's death, still wonders, "Why Bob?" They adored each other. The question is evident in my hairdresser Pat's beautiful black eyes as she watches Ronnie die from throat cancer. It's bound to be ringing in Janet's ears now that Jim is gone. At the memorial service I heard his fishing buddy Craig ask the question, "Why Jim? Look at all the people he counseled . . . and his first book was just published! . . . Why?"

I could see the question in my friend Betsy's eyes as she drifted in and out of consciousness after her diseased stomach was removed, and again even more intensely at Dana's wedding shower, when it occurred to her she may not be around for her daughter Sara's high school graduation, much less her wedding.

A day or two after my mastectomy, a strikingly beautiful woman with a halo of vivid red hair entered my hospital room. She introduced herself as Michelle, a friend of a friend, and gently described her own battle with breast cancer. "You know, Sue, it was terrible to go through; but now as I look back, I believe I was *privileged* to have had this experience."

Privileged? I thought. *What a strange thing to say.* Michelle explained that her life had been in turmoil before this overwhelming interference but that the experience had changed everything. She described a new and vital relationship with God, a deeper love for her family, and a delight for life never before experienced.

A better, more sensitive and compassionate person maybe, but privileged? I thought. *No way!*

Different people seem to have different viewpoints on the *why me?* question. My friend George Volkert is in property development. There are big red signs all over parts of Nashville that say "Southeast Venture." George owns that company. Several years ago my company was engaged to produce a high-impact media show for the visitors' center at SEV headquarters. When I met George, I was impressed! The walls and plants and draperies were impressed with George! He had the biggest, friendliest smile you can imagine, and appeared to be one of those people who knows exactly what he wants when he wants it—a no-grass-growing-under-his-feet type man.

After my work was finished, I lost track of George, but each time I passed a big red sign, I thought about him. Then one day someone asked, "Did you hear about George Volkert? Poor ol' George, he has leukemia . . . doesn't look too good!" Somehow I couldn't imagine George slowing down, even for a freight train. I prayed a prayer and sent a note. Last week I heard from him. He called me at the office, and we talked for almost an hour. He's in remission and is doing great.

"What do you make of it, George? Do you ever ask *why me?*" I was curious about this dynamo of a businessman.

"Sure have." I could picture George rolling back in his executive chair and putting his feet on his big executive-size desk. ". . . but ya know, Sue, I never thought *why me* when I got tackled in football and got the daylights knocked out of me. You don't go around sayin' *why me* when you're playin' for Georgia Tech, at least not out loud; and believe me you gotta have a whole different level of tolerance for pain when you're playin' for Georgia Tech. You get knocked down and you get hurt, but you don't stay down. You get up and play again."

"What'dja learn George?" I asked.

"My priorities have changed. I'm enjoying my family more. And you know what really means a lot to me? I've heard from people I hadn't thought of in thirty-five years, people who followed my football career when I was younger. I learned that people care." We chatted for a while and, unlike our first meeting, were relaxed and laid back. There wasn't some urgency to single-handedly conquer the world in the next ten minutes on either of our parts. "One more thing, Sue," he said in his most philosophic voice, "I think about the Lord more, and I think when the Lord is ready to take us, He'll take us. I don't worry anymore about things I can't control."

It seems to me that the great cause and effect ratio present in most people who have experienced a brush with death is an awakening or renewing of the awareness of God's presence in their lives. If the desire for God's presence wasn't there in the first place, often there is a first-time experience of *finding* God. One person I know, a good ol' boy type who had cancer expressed it well when he said, "I got religion, real fast and real good!"

It was certainly true for me. It's difficult for me to believe we are moving through life randomly, that it is luck or chance or that it's simply "written in the stars." It's equally hard for me to think that God created us and walked away. During my year of chemotherapy, when I wasn't sure whether I would die, it became important for me to sort myth from truth in regard to my personal faith.

I came to see that God wasn't nearly as complicated as I had once thought Him to be. In fact, it became easy for me to think of Him as a loving parent who sees the big picture, just as Wayne and I saw the big picture for our children when they were young and immature. It would have been tempting to keep them locked up in an environmental bubble like those used for children with no immune system. Instead, we made decisions we felt would keep them safe, and we made decisions we thought would make them wise. There were always things they not only questioned, but also didn't have the capacity to understand.

Often bad things happened to our children that we didn't cause, yet we tried to use those negative things for their good. We spent a great deal of time and energy protecting them from bad things, and yet some of their most painful experiences taught them the most valuable lessons.

I have no trouble at all believing that the heavenly Parent took a negative thing like cancer and used it for good. I learned a Bible verse at summer camp one year that said, "All things work together for good to those who love God" (Rom. 8:28).

My painful experience taught me new things about my husband: first of all how much he loves me and that I can count on him to take care of me. In fact, I have no doubt he would fix me his cure-all tomato soup night after night till the end of time, if need be. I don't want him to know it, but one of the reasons I got well so quickly was that I was pretty tired of that soup!

Family history was preserved because of my life-threatening illness. The stack of photo albums gets higher, and stories are repeated over and over so as to burn them into the minds of my children, my brothers, and their families.

I've learned to nurture friendships. I've come to understand and care about the hurts of others and find time to visit and send cards, something I never did before.

When my problems slowed me down enough to let it sink in, I discovered that God was as close as I allowed Him to be. I could actually feel His presence. When my prayers didn't seem to be getting any higher than the ceiling fan, I realized my friends were there waiting to take over for me. They were praying *for* me. I began to count on those prayers and I began to respond to God's *nudges*—when He brought someone to my mind—to pray for others.

Having cancer and having to go through a year of treatment may not have been a *privilege*, and I wouldn't wish it to happen to anyone else, but it makes me stop and ask, "Why not me?" My perspective has changed on almost everything: family, friendship, reunions, my Christian faith, sunsets, and porpoise shows.

After realizing that God was *there* and that He wasn't as complicated as I'd thought, the next thing I discovered was that there are answers to all of life's dilemmas in Scripture. Sometimes we aren't even aware they are there until we need them. I was a tape recorder that could be turned on and off; push my button and I could turn on the verse that speaks of a "peace . . . which surpasses all understanding" (Phil. 4:7). One day in a hospital room, the reality of those words sank in.

Two weeks before Bob died, he was still managing, with Peggy's help, to get to the sink to shave, brush his teeth, and comb his hair. It was a chore. Bob was so weak that when Peggy got him in front of the mirror, she would have to brace him there with her body. One day their eyes caught in the mirror, and tears came. "Bob, have you been talkin' to the Lord this morning?" Peggy said. Bob nodded. "Bob, did you ask him, *Why you? Why us?*" Bob nodded again. "What did He say?"

"He said, 'Ah, Bob when you get to the place where you'll know the answer, the question isn't going to matter.' "

The third thing I learned (I should have learned it long ago—it's just that it seemed so far down the road) is that life here on earth isn't the end. The reality has finally sunk in. I believe that because I have chosen to be a follower of Jesus Christ, someday I'll arrive at that *place* Bob referred to. The Scripture I learned as a child, "Today shalt thou be with me in paradise" (Luke 23:43 KJV), has a deep and passionate meaning for me and is a concept that now seems like a possibility. Singing the old gospel song, "There's Going to Be a Meeting in the Air," that we sang with my parents and sang again after Dana's wedding, creates in me a strangely appealing longing.

To me, the original party girl, it means that God is planning a wingdinger of a party, and I'll be there! There will be decorations, food, and a band—or at least the heavenly equivalent. There will be family and friends, and it will go on forever! There's something else I know. It will be *so beautiful!* My daddy saw it that day so long ago, and he told me it was so.

"When can I say I'm cured?" I asked Dr. Solomon not long ago. "Is ten years the magic number?"

"When you die of natural causes," he replied. Not *if,* but *when!* Aunt Annie said it best: "It'll get you. Sure as shootin', it'll get you!" Even as I frantically shuffled through the family keepsakes at the time of Mother's death and tried to connect with the ancestors that shaped my life, I knew *beyond the shadow of a doubt* that someday I would join them in death, and that soon after, the signposts of my own life would be reduced to a scrapbook, a few keepsakes, and a brass box full of pictures.

I *will* die. Someday I may get a bad report that cancer cells have once again invaded my body. Perhaps I'll be hit by a car or die of "natural causes." When that day comes, I can wholeheartedly say, "Let the party begin!"

> I used to think
> loving life so greatly
> that to die would be like
> leaving the party before the end.

> But now I know that the party is really happening
>   somewhere else,
> that the light and the music escaping in snatches
> to make the pulse beat faster and the tempo quicken
>   comes from another place.

> And I know too
> that when I get there,

the music and the love and the praise
will belong to Him,
and the music will never end.

Author unknown
(and may already be at the party!)

Rap

I've promised my friends at the American Cancer Society and the National Cancer Institute that whenever I speak or write I'll call attention to breast health. Because I'm a video producer, I'm always looking for a new way to tell an old story. I've used rap music to introduce a new product, for a training film, and for the finale at a large convention. Clap your hands to an imaginary drumbeat, think mean, and read

This rap's about a subject not often discussed
Self-breast examination, you know it's a must!
You bettah listen to us, we're here to crusade
We're the breast self-examination brigade.

What are our credentials? Why're we campaignin'?
Well, we've all had cancer, so we know what we're sayin'
We're gonna tell you the facts. We're gonna tell you the rules
So listen real close now. Don't be fools!

Ready?

When you're in the shower or the tub
Make this routine a part of your scrub
Lather your hands and examine your breasts
With soap on your hands you can feel them best.

Now stand before the mirror. Don't rush!
Get acquainted with your body. Don't blush!
First arms at your side; then high in the air
Make sure there are no discrepancies there.

Then raise your arms horizontally,
Check yourself for a visual abnormality
Ch-ch-check yourself for abnormality!

Next lie on your back, left hand behind your head
Use your right hand to check with fingers outspread
(Use a circular motion, a c-c-circular motion.)
You're looking for lumps that might be hid.
Now using your left hand, repeat what you just did.
(with a circular motion, a c-c-circular motion.)

Take care of your body, it's the only one you got.
Have regular mammograms; stay close to your doc!
Till we can put cancer in the past tense
You gotta go usin' a little bit'a horse sense.

So be wise, be intelligent, be realistic
Just follow these rules, don't be a statistic
Follow these rules. D-D-D-Don't be a statistic!

(copyright 1993, Dynamic Media, Inc.)

HOTLINE NUMBERS

* Alive Hospice
  Check your local directory
* American Cancer Society
  Volunteer organization with divisions in all major cities in the
  United States. The hotline number will connect you with an ACS
  chapter near you. (800) ACS-2345 or write: 90 Park Avenue,
  New York, New York 10016.
* ASPRS (American Society of Plastic and Reconstructive Sur-
  geons, Inc.)
  Free referral service to board certified plastic surgeons.
  (800) 635-0635 or write: 444 East Algonquin Road, Arlington
  Heights, Illinois 60005-4664.
* Cancer Information Service
  Accurate, personalized answers to your cancer-related questions.
  (800) 4-CANCER.
* Cansurmount
  Provides patient and family support services. Tries to match a vol-
  unteer with a patient. Write in care of the American Cancer Soci-
  ety: 90 Park Avenue, New York, New York 10016.
* The Institute for Aesthetic and Reconstructive Surgery
  Serves as a nationwide resource facility for educational informa-
  tion or assistance. (800) 328-4277.
* Look Good, Feel Better
  Learn to cope with the changes in your appearance due to cancer
  treatment from professionally trained makeup artists and hair
  consultants. Contact your local ACS chapter for more informa-
  tion.
* National Cancer Institute
  To find a physician or more information about cancer.
  (800) 4-CANCER.
* Reach to Recovery
  Provides assistance to women with breast cancer. Write in care of
  ACS: 90 Park Avenue, New York, New York 10016 or contact
  your local ACS chapter.
* Y-ME
  Support for women with breast cancer, including bimonthly

newsletters. (800) 221-2141 or write: 18220 Harwood Avenue, Homewood, Illinois 60430.

Emotional support groups are available in many cities throughout the United States. Call the American Cancer Society for groups in your area.